S0-AHN-784

**Pioneers**

# JONAS SALK

rourke biographies

## Pioneers

# JONAS SALK

*by*
**MICHAEL TOMLINSON**



Rourke Publications, Inc.
Vero Beach, Florida 32964

∞ The paper used in this book conforms to the American National Standard for Permanence of Paper for Printed Library Materials, Z39.48-1984.

**Library of Congress Cataloging-in-Publication Data**
Tomlinson, Michael, 1967-
Jonas Salk / written by Michael Tomlinson.
p. cm. — (Rourke biographies. Pioneers)
Includes bibliographical references and index.
Summary: A biography of the scientist and humanitarian who discovered the vaccine for polio, a disease which crippled many people in the early part of the century.
ISBN 0-86625-495-1 (alk. paper)
1. Salk, Jonas, 1914- —Juvenile literature. 2. Virologists—United States—Biography—Juvenile literature. 3. Poliomyelitis vaccine—History—Juvenile literature. [1. Salk, Jonas, 1914- . 2. Scientists. 3. Poliomyelitis vaccine.] I. Title. II. Series.
QR31.S25T66 1993
610′.92—dc20
[B] 92-46284
CIP
AC



PRINTED IN THE UNITED STATES OF AMERICA

# Contents

# Color Illustrations

**Pioneers**

---

# JONAS SALK

# Chapter 1

# Science with a Human Face

It is impossible to talk about Dr. Jonas Salk and not mention the disease poliomyelitis, or polio. In the 1950's polio was the most feared disease in the public's mind, much as AIDS is today. Dr. Salk was the first person to find a vaccine for the deadly polio virus, which crippled and killed thousands. Furthermore, Dr. Salk was able to develop his vaccine at least ten years faster than most people thought possible, saving countless lives. The organization and imagination with which he attacked polio were truly inspired. Yet just as remarkable as his scientific achievements are the humanitarian qualities that Dr. Salk has consistently brought to his work.

In 1955, the most popular news show on television was called "See It Now," hosted by the first famous television newscaster, Edward Murrow. On Tuesday, April 12, 1955, viewers tuned in to Murrow's "See It Now" in even greater numbers than usual. That night Dr. Jonas Salk was the special guest. Earlier that day he had announced that his laboratory had created a successful vaccine for polio. Families across the country wanted to see the man who had saved them from a frightening disease that could put them in an iron lung or even kill them—a disease that caused people to worry so much that they would stay inside on the hottest days of summer for fear that they might be the next victim.

A tall, thin man with glasses, Salk closely resembled the popular image of the scientist as portrayed in movies. In the interview, he patiently explained how his vaccine worked, and how it would eventually bring about the end of the polio threat. Murrow then asked Dr. Salk who owned the patent for the

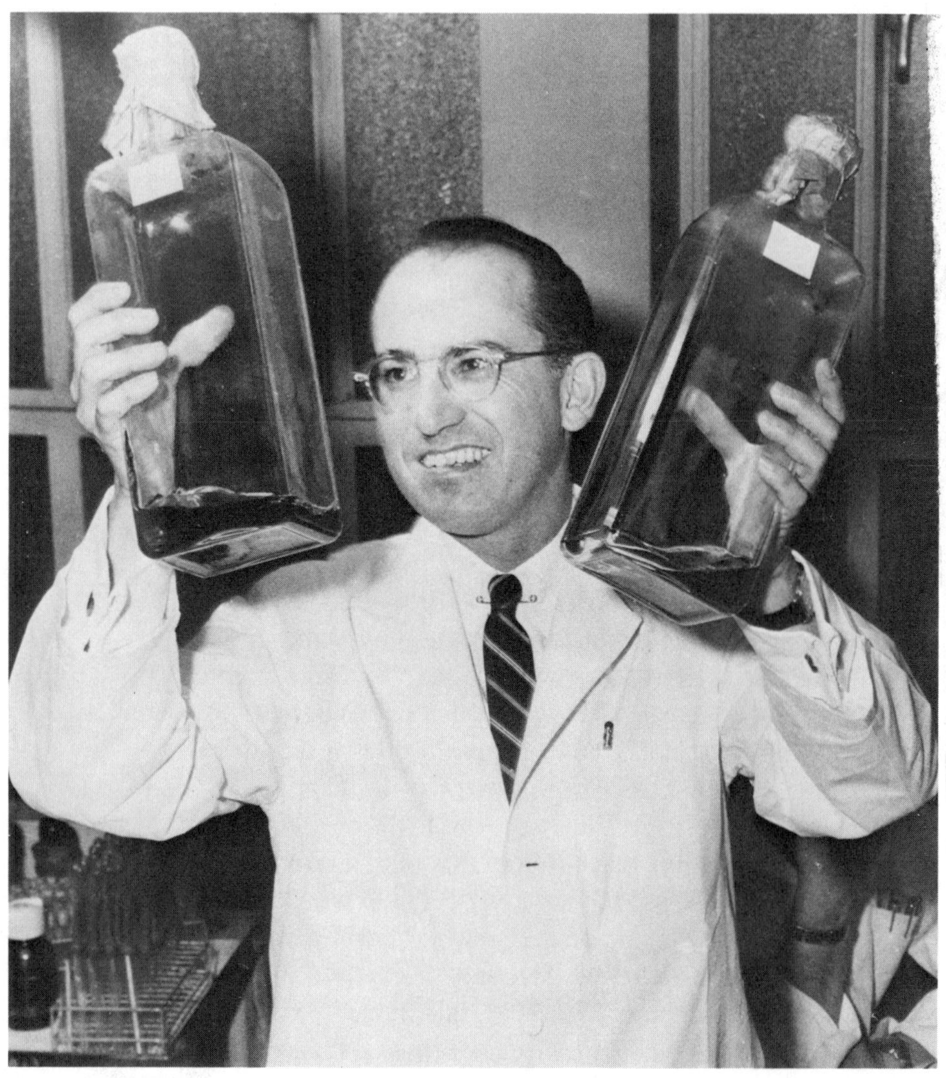

*Jonas Salk holding two bottles containing a culture used to grow the polio vaccine.* (AP/ Wide World Photos)

vaccine. It was obvious that whoever owned the vaccine would make lots of money. Every person in the United States and the rest of the world was susceptible to polio, and all people would, of course, want to receive the vaccine. Dr. Salk thought for only a second before he answered. The people owned the patent, he said. "There is no patent. Could you patent the sun?" Dr. Salk wanted people to be safe and healthy, and was not concerned with making a profit from his work. The vaccine was his gift to the people.

## A Global Outlook

Dr. Salk is a scientific pioneer, but he is perhaps best described as a great humanitarian. In all his varied projects his underlying goal has always been to look for a way to better the human condition. Dr. Salk has said that the reward for a job well done is that you get to do more work. He has made this statement true in his own life, but not without overcoming many challenges. Even though Dr. Salk's work in the laboratory, turning ideas into usable medicines, has been very practical and successful, he has had to break new ground in many other ways.

Dr. Salk's appearance on "See It Now" is a good example. Dr. Salk is one of a handful of scientists who have become media figures and taken on the responsibility of making science a public issue, something to which the common person must pay attention. In the past, scientific ideas and projects often did not have quick or specific applications in everyday life. Thus, when the vaccine that Dr. Salk created was distributed to millions of people in 1955, he was covering new ground not only by curing a disease but also by making science accessible to the average person.

Today we are used to seeing space-shuttle astronauts or AIDS researchers on television and in newspapers. We see the application of scientific discoveries in satellites, microwave

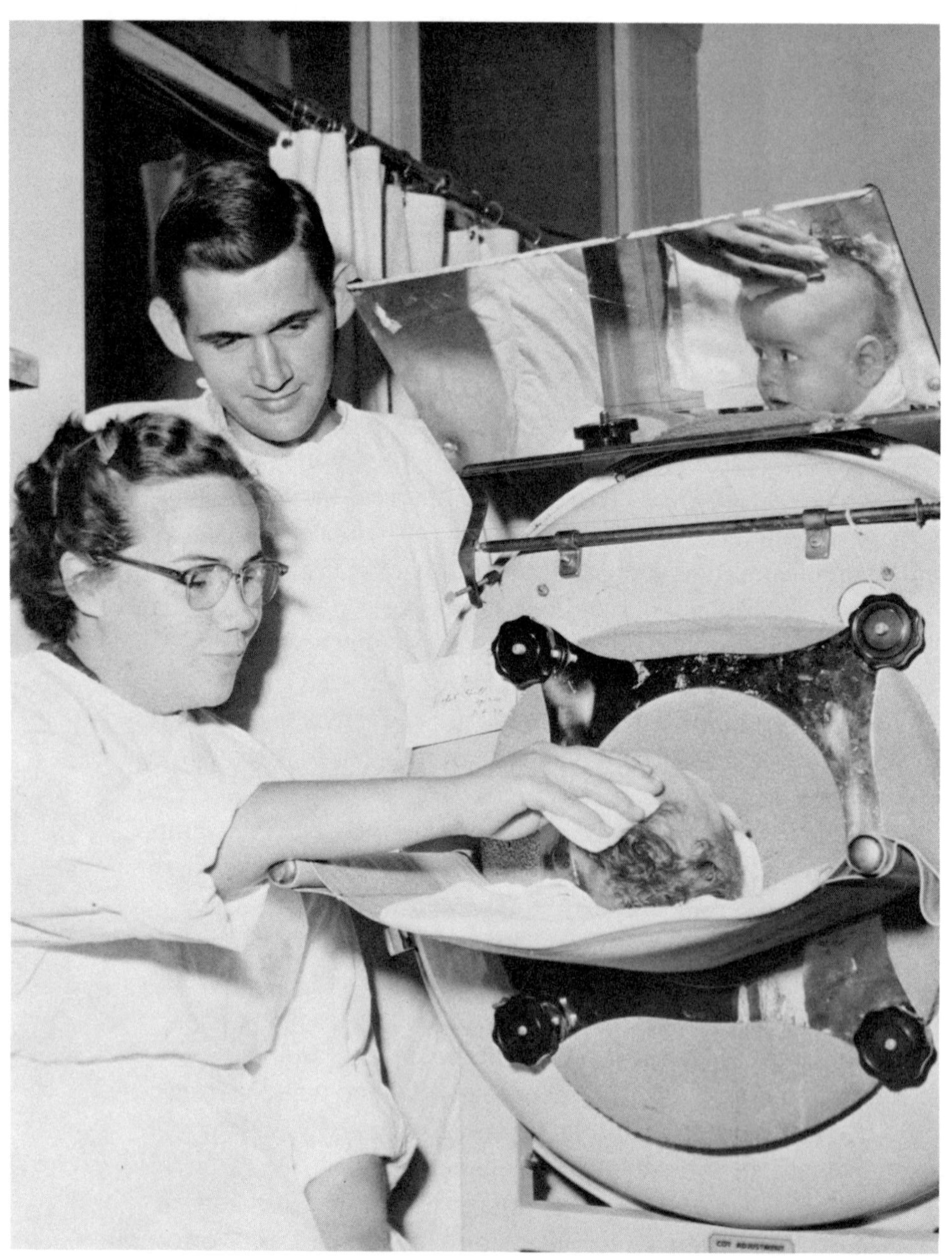

*Before the Salk vaccine: an eleven-week-old polio victim.* (AP/Wide World Photos)

ovens, and countless other features of everyday life. Dr. Salk was a pioneer in increasing public awareness of science and its enormous impact on our lives. At the same time, Dr. Salk was a pioneer for other scientists who were not used to doing their research in the public eye and often didn't think of ways their work could be used immediately to help people.

Dr. Salk has always been a scientist who sees his work and all aspects of human existence as connected. This broad way of looking at things, a global approach, is particularly important today. As a result of the tremendous increase in the world's population and the pressure this growth puts on the environment, as well as the increased speed of communication and travel between all parts of the world, events truly are interconnected as never before. Regional wars, famines, and other such tragedies can be prevented only if people throughout the world adopt a global outlook, as Dr. Salk has done.

Your life has been made better by the hard work of Dr. Salk and the scientists who worked with him to find vaccines for the polio virus. Today children in the United States and other developed countries grow up never having heard of polio. It is easy to take for granted this freedom from the threat of polio, but ask someone who grew up before 1955 about the disease and the fear and suffering it caused. Then you will begin to appreciate the important achievements of Dr. Jonas Salk and others like him who have devoted their lives to understanding the workings of the world's smallest creatures and how they fit into the big picture so that we all can live a healthier life.

## Polio

*The polio virus has existed for a very long time—exactly how long, nobody knows—but only in the twentieth century did it become an epidemic disease. In earlier times, polio (though not identified as such) had taken the form of a common and relatively mild childhood disease. Early exposure to the disease resulted in lifetime immunity. Modern sanitation, however, made the polio virus much less common and at the same time more deadly, since many people had not developed an immunity against it.*

*Like AIDS, polio puzzled scientists when it first appeared. They were perplexed by the fact that the disease struck people in suburbs and upper-class neighborhoods, where nutrition and sanitation were excellent, as well as in crowded tenements.*

*Epidemics occurred only in the summer; the first large epidemic occurred in 1916. Victims typically had the symptoms of a common cold—headache and a slight fever. After several days, most people recovered, but the worst cases became paralyzed without warning after a couple of days. The virus attacked the parts of the nervous system that control muscles; in fatal cases, the muscles in the lungs were paralyzed, resulting in suffocation. Some victims were kept alive in huge metal respirators. Only a patient's head stuck out of these machines, which were called iron lungs.*

*As treatments and physical therapy improved, fewer cases caused permanent paralysis, but the disease continued to take its toll until Dr. Salk and, later, Dr. Albert Sabin developed effective vaccines.*

# Chapter 2

# The Long, Hard Climb

Jonas Salk was born on October 28, 1914, in New York City. To understand how he became a medical researcher and developed the great compassion he would show in all his work, we need to look first at his parents, grandparents, and great-grandparents and their Russian Jewish culture. This culture deeply influenced the way Jonas Salk was brought up and the way he learned to see the world.

## Russian Jewish Culture

Historically, Jews all over the world—especially in Europe—have been treated with prejudice. Anti-Semitism, or prejudice against Jews, has taken many forms, ranging from discriminatory laws to violent persecution. In the 1930's and 1940's under Adolf Hitler, Germany and its allies murdered more than six million Jewish men, women, and children. This orgy of killing had deep roots in European history.

Because they were different from the Christian majority in Eastern European countries such as Russia, Poland, and Hungary, the Jews were forced to live apart in villages called shtetls or in restricted areas in cities, called ghettos. Moreover, Jews were not allowed to own land. Despite persecution, many Jews attained success. At a time when relatively few people knew how to read, write, and do mathematics, Jews were able to fill jobs that required those skills.

Education and learning have always played a central role in Jewish culture. In traditional Jewish culture, study was largely devoted to the Torah: the Jewish Scripture and the enormous body of commentary that had grown around it. By the

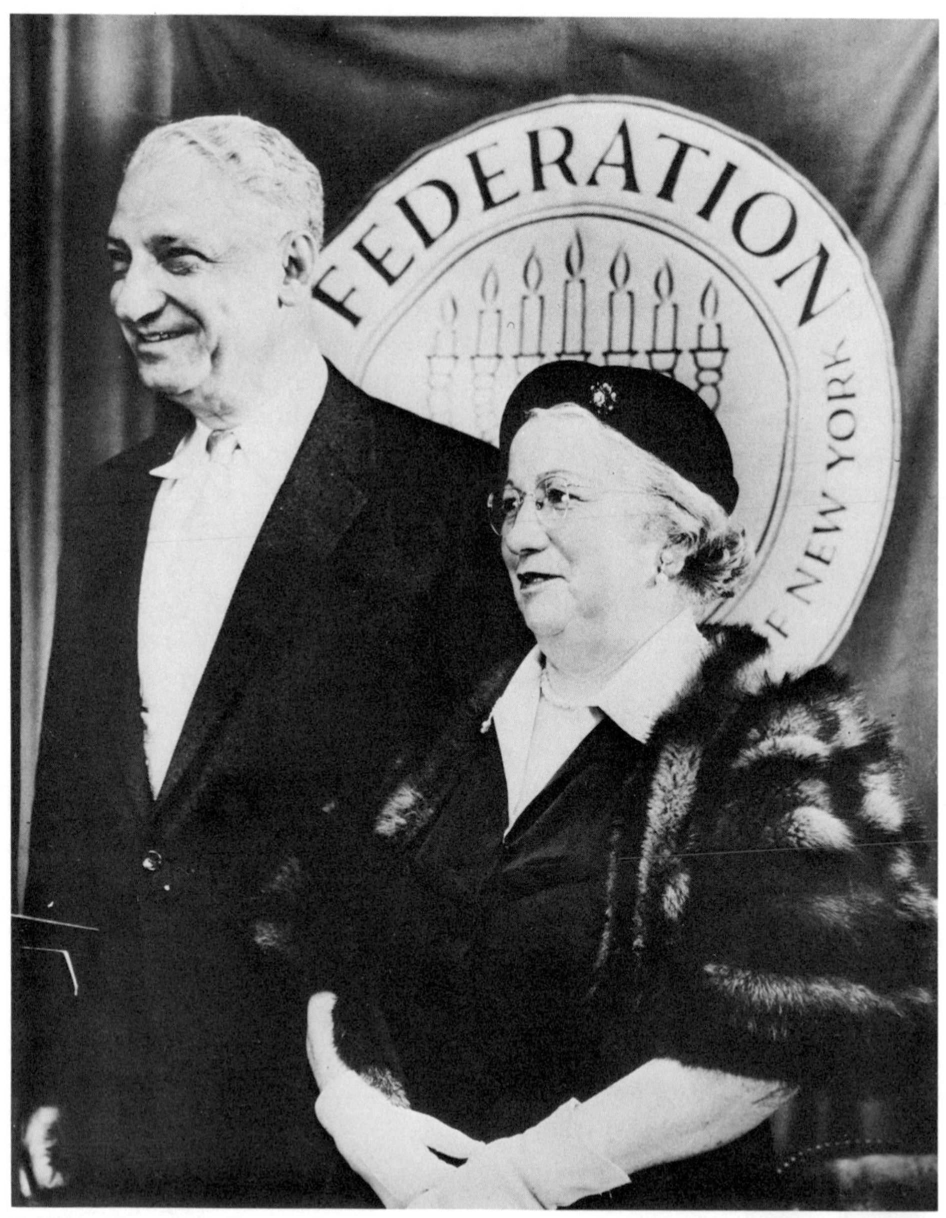


*Salk's mother and father, receiving a citation in 1955 honoring them as "Jewish Parents of the Year."* (AP/Wide World Photos)

nineteenth century, however, many Jews had begun to study secular subjects. An extraordinary number of the leading figures in modern science have been Jewish—including, most notably, Albert Einstein. This was the tradition that nurtured Jonas Salk.

Another aspect of Jewish culture that shaped Jonas Salk's life was the close sense of community and charity that he experienced as a youth. Since they were attacked on all sides, Jews looked out for and helped everyone in their community who was in need. Salk was able to take this sense of obligation to the community—which exists in all cultures, but was particularly strong in the persecuted Jewish culture—and broaden it to all of humankind.

Living in communities separate from the mainstream, the only person the Russian Jewish grandparents of Jonas Salk saw who was on equal footing in all communities, rich and poor, Christian and Jewish, was the doctor. Doctors were learned and universally respected; their skills were always in demand, and they generally enjoyed financial security. These attributes, as well as the intrinsic value of someone who could heal and help the injured and ill, ensured that the medical profession would be highly regarded—probably the most highly regarded—among Eastern European Jews who immigrated to the United States.

In the late nineteenth century, times were hard in Russia. Without any justification, many Russian people blamed the Jews for their problems. Mobs, acting with the support of the government, killed many Jews and burned their homes and belongings. This was the death of hope for a good life in Europe for many Russian Jews. Those who could decided to cross the Atlantic Ocean to the United States and start over. Jonas Salk's parents, Daniel and Dolly, were among these immigrants. Naturally, they brought with them the culture and ideas of their homeland. They also brought with them a strong desire that their children take advantage of the opportunities for advancement that the United States offered.

## The Lower East Side

Certainly, things were not easy for immigrants such as Salk's parents. They arrived in New York at the turn of the century with little money and only the belongings they could carry. To make life even harder, they spoke very little English or none at all and knew very little about the laws, culture, and customs of the country they had just entered. Most Eastern European Jews first settled in the slums of New York's Lower East Side.

In some ways the horrors of the Lower East Side in 1900 were worse than anything to be found in the inner-city slums of America in the 1990's. That the people who lived there were not completely demoralized is a sign of their cultural and personal strength of character. A teenage boy or girl in the Lower East Side would probably awake long before dawn in a one-room apartment with one window, no running water, and a toilet that was down the hall and shared by everyone on the floor. Around the room would sleep six or seven siblings, the mother and father, and perhaps one or two boarders, usually young men who helped pay the rent in exchange for floor space. Privacy was nonexistent.

Food was expensive and not always of good quality; families ate what they could on the pitifully low wages they were paid for working up to sixteen hours a day at the garment factory sweatshops that were the primary employers in the area. The teenagers would go to school, if they were lucky, and work in the factories if they were needed. Either way, work assembling clothes was often brought home, and the whole family would gather around and sew in their spare minutes to make extra money. The streets outside were often crowded to a standstill with peddlers and carts of wares at almost any hour.

Many immigrant families worked ceaselessly to get ahead so that their children would have the opportunities they did not have. This work ethic was passed on to their children. Even so, the Russian Jews found that their old enemy, anti-Semitism, had followed them in the new country. When they tried to move to some neighborhoods, they were told that they were not welcome. They were discriminated against in business dealings, in schools, and in courts of law. Still, there were opportunities for change—opportunities that had brought the Russian Jews to the United States in the first place.

As an ethnic and cultural group, the immigrant Jews of New York turned to education to break down the barriers that held them back. The Lower East Side boasted more schools than perhaps any other slum neighborhood in history. There were newspapers that focused exclusively on the Lower East Side and an active and well-attended theater scene. In the neighborhood coffee shops, lively intellectual conversations took place and gave rise to many of the first labor unions in New York. Schools for orphans and other charities were set up to help the many needy people. Activities of this kind could be found among other immigrant groups, but they were especially prominent in the Jewish Lower East Side.

Jonas Salk was born into this culture and society. There is no doubt that he was moved by the suffering and poverty he saw around him in his youth and that he heard about through his parents. Equally important was the energy and work ethic of the community. Faced with huge problems, the community that Salk was born into sought to make immediate and humanitarian changes through their hard work and courage. The work of Jonas Salk is his own, but he is also a product of the immigrant Jewish culture of his youth.

## The Salk Family

Soon after Jonas Salk's birth, his parents had saved enough

money to move to a slightly nicer neighborhood in East Harlem. In time, their savings increased further, and the Salks moved to Brooklyn, where many other families who had started out in the slums of the Lower East Side made their home.

Salk was expected to do well in school because of his parents' sacrifices, and he did not disappoint them. He was accepted into Townsand Harris High School, an accelerated school, at the age of twelve; at fifteen, he began studies at the College of the City of New York (CCNY). At a time when many colleges would not accept Jewish students or strictly limited their admission, and cost prevented many children of immigrants from even thinking about college, CCNY was an amazing opportunity, and Salk took advantage of it fully.

Daniel and Dolly Salk had the same expectations for their two younger sons, Herman and Lee, as they did for Jonas. They were not disappointed by any of their sons. Both Herman and Lee developed the same work ethic and humanitarian ideals that inspired Jonas.

Herman Salk became a veterinarian. For a time, his practice included caring for the animals used in Jonas' lab. Later he served on United Nations food and health committees as a livestock and agricultural consultant. Although Herman was not in the public eye as his brothers were, his work was valuable and important.

Lee Salk achieved fame nearly equal to Jonas' through his work in child psychology. He first gained widespread notice for research showing that babies are calmer when they can hear a heartbeat. He then turned to more theoretical aspects of psychology, focusing on child-rearing and family relations. Lee was able to deal with universal issues in a clear, accessible way; several of his books, such as *What Every Child Would Like His Parents to Know* and *My Father, My Son: Intimate Relationships*, became best-sellers. In the 1970's, Lee became a familiar face on the "Today" show and "Good Morning, America," where he gave family counseling advice. He also had a column in *McCall's* magazine until his death in 1992.

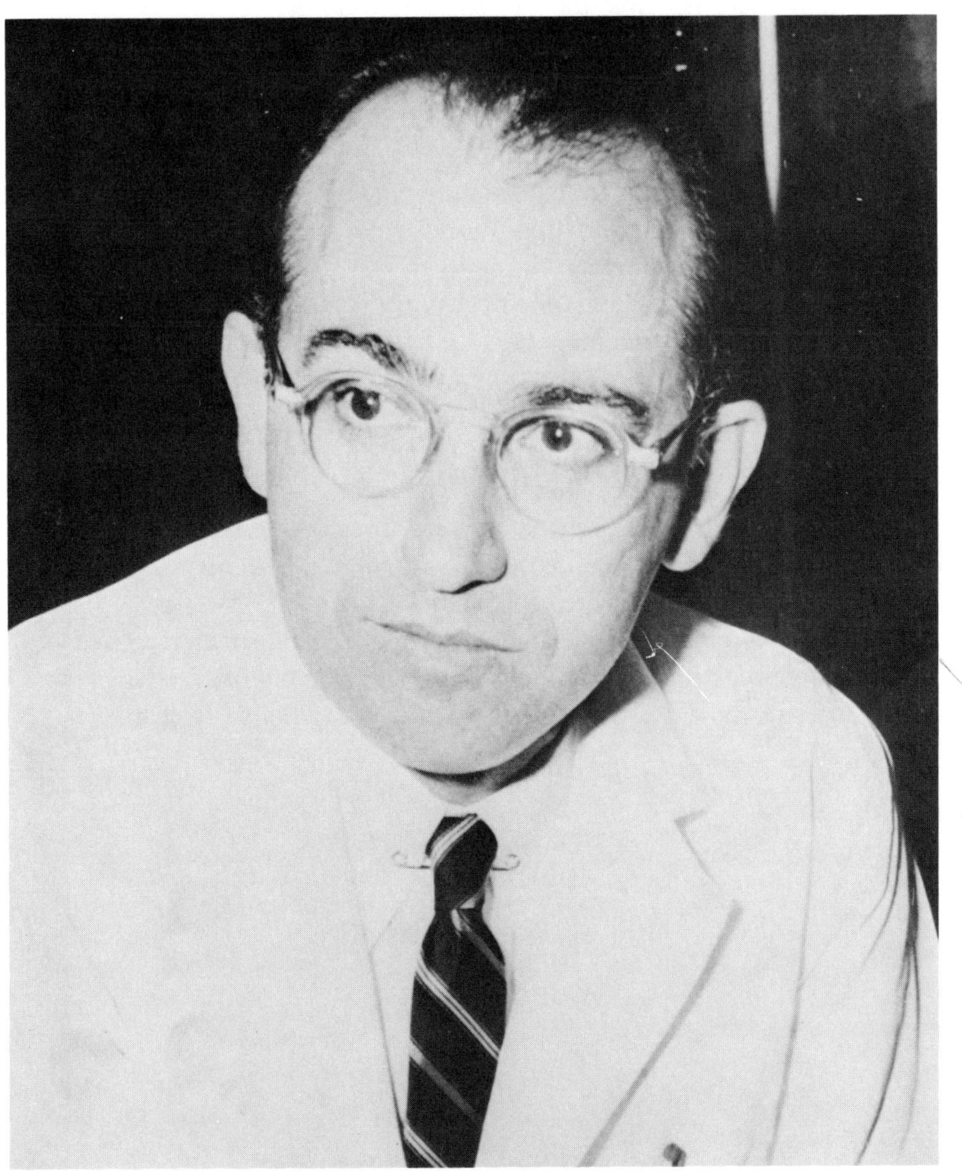

*Salk in 1955.* (AP/Wide World Photos)

## The Great Depression

When Jonas Salk began college, an event occurred that would affect his generation profoundly. In 1929, the stock market crashed, and the United States plunged into the Great Depression. For the next ten years, the country suffered the most widespread and lasting general poverty it had ever seen. In that time, the poverty that had previously been confined to the slums became a concern for everyone. Businesses folded, banks were unable to pay out money people had saved, and droughts killed farm crops. Working people across the country were put on the streets. Going to classes, Salk would surely have passed a veteran of World War I standing on a corner selling apples for a nickel apiece to survive. Going to a library, he was surely asked by an unemployed person, "Brother, can you spare a dime?"

Many people who lived through the Great Depression came out of it with a sense that there was great suffering in America and throughout the world, and something had to be done to ease it. The combination of growing up in the immigrant Russian Jewish culture of New York, the great drive to succeed that his parents gave him, and living through the Great Depression no doubt influenced Jonas Salk to work on the projects he did and to pursue them with such great intensity.

# Chapter 3

# Learning to Ask Why

Jonas Salk cut his teeth in the medical and scientific world between 1936 and 1947. In this period he went through medical school and started on the path of medical research that he would follow for the rest of his life. During this time he also learned that the questioning of accepted beliefs is not always welcomed, even in the scientific community. He became self-sufficient, and his independent nature became evident. Except for a loan his parents took out in his first year of medical school, he financed his entire schooling himself, through grants he was awarded in recognition of his hard work and through jobs on the side.

## Viruses and Vaccines

In 1936, in his second year of medical school at CCNY, Salk was exposed to a set of ideas that would set him on the course to conquering polio fifteen years later. In a class on bacteriology, the study of microscopic organisms called bacteria and the diseases they cause, he was taught that people could be made immune to bacterial diseases by inoculation with a vaccine. A vaccine is made by isolating the infecting bacteria in a test tube and then killing them so that they are no longer infectious but still look like they are alive to the body's immune system. A person is then injected with these killed bacteria to make the body's immune system react as if the body was being attacked by the disease.

In other words, vaccination tricks the body into developing protection against an infection that does not exist. If that disease ever does attack the body, the body's immune system can "remember" the invading bacteria and produce specific antibodies, cells that kill the intruder, and stop the disease before it starts. A vaccine tells your body how to react to a disease before you ever get it.

Later, in a class on virology, the study of viruses and the diseases they cause, Salk was told that immunity to diseases caused by viruses could only be attained if the patient was infected with a weakened, but still live virus, referred to by virologists as an *attenuated* virus. Patients vaccinated with an attenuated virus actually experience a mild form of the disease, but the immune system is easily able to conquer the infection, after which the body is immune to future attacks by the virus. The risk of this method is that the mild infection caused by the vaccination can develop into the full-blown disease. Nevertheless, Salk and his fellow-students were told, this risk was unavoidable.

Many years later, in an interview with *Discovery* magazine, Salk would recall the questions that came to his mind in medical school: "I asked, 'Why should this be true of a virus [but not true of bacteria]?' and my teachers answered 'Because.' That's no answer. So I tried to put myself in the place of the virus, and the immune system, and see how they would behave and why. I began to do this whenever I had to deal with things that seemed paradoxical." Salk's observational skills and his ability to question accepted notions were awakened by this paradox and became the cornerstone of his thinking.

## Finding a Mentor

In medical school Salk became more and more interested in problems in the research side of medicine. His family and friends did not understand why he would give up the chance to make a good living as a practicing doctor, but after his second year of medical school, when he received a fellowship to

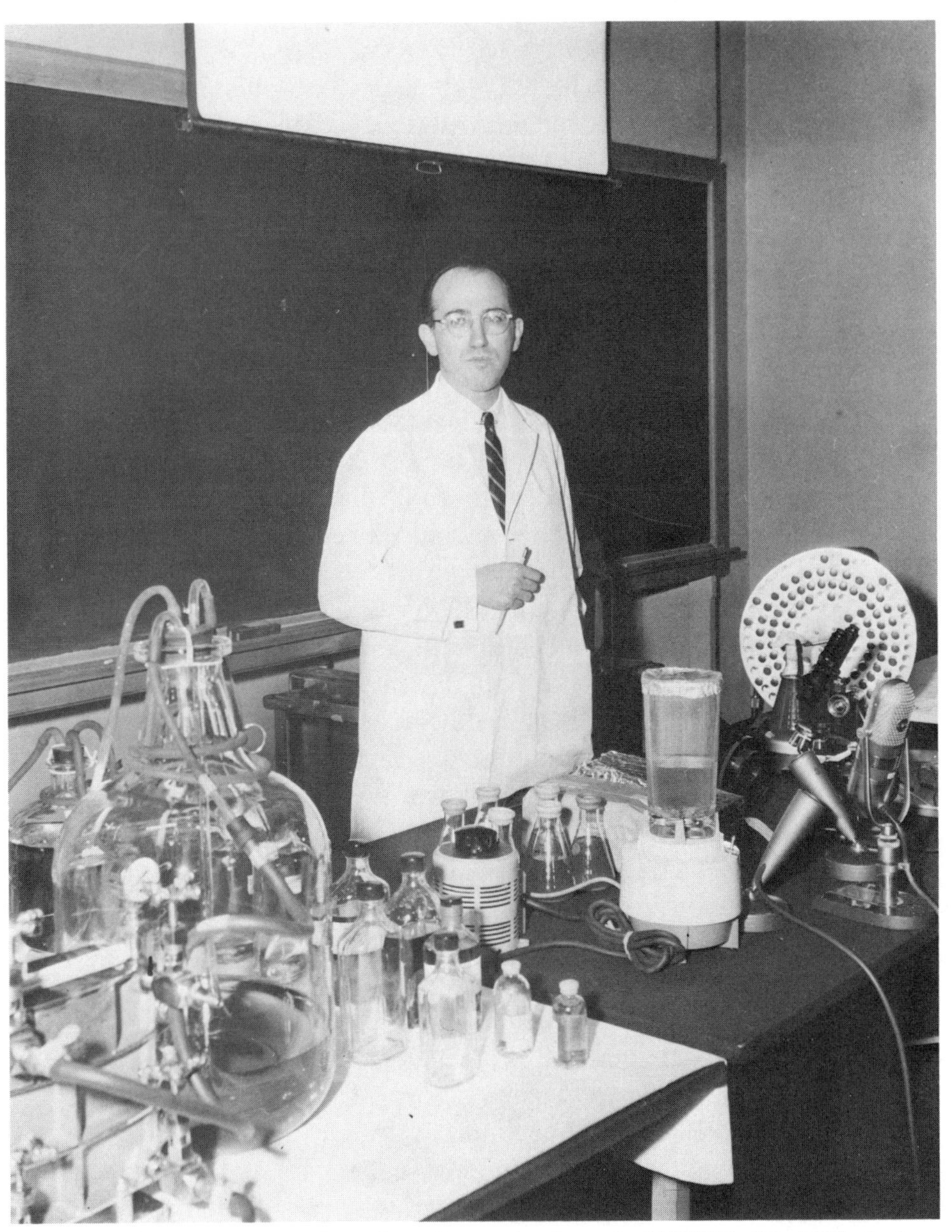

*Salk explains to reporters how the polio vaccine is made.* (AP/Wide World Photos)

spend a year in special studies of biochemistry, they saw that it was an area in which he was truly talented. By his final year in medical school, Salk had decided to devote himself to research. He arranged to do his independent senior work with Dr. Thomas Francis, a respected virologist, who was doing work on influenza viruses at the University of New York.

It was a lucky meeting for both men. Dr. Francis was an exacting and unimpeachable researcher who sported a trim mustache and had a wry sense of humor. He was also one of the few virologists who believed that viral diseases could be prevented by killed-virus vaccines. Salk saw Francis as someone who could teach him a great deal and who was sympathetic to ideas he already had, while Francis found in Salk a skilled young lab technician who could think independently.

Francis immediately put Salk to work helping him with his research on a vaccine for influenza, a flu virus. He had Salk remove influenza viruses from infected mice's lungs, kill the viruses with intense ultraviolet light, and then test the viruses to see if they had any value for a vaccine. The process didn't yield favorable results, but Salk was in seventh heaven because he was working in the area of his interest. With the aid of Francis, he was able to publish his first scientific paper, a major step toward becoming an established researcher. Salk was not designing his own experiments, his ultimate goal, but he was learning the skills that would allow him to work independently in the future.

Salk's elation was heightened at this time because he was courting his first wife, Donna Lindsay. Donna was an idealistic social worker fresh out of Smith College, and the young couple found that their excitement in their work was surpassed only by their excitement about each other. In 1939 they became engaged, and they were married the following year.

## Internship at Mt. Sinai

All medical students are required to work at internships in hospitals before they can become full M.D.s. In March, 1940, Salk had to leave Dr. Francis' research team and intern at the emergency ward of Mt. Sinai Hospital in New York City, one of the most distinguished hospitals in the United States. Although Salk would rather have continued working on basic research, it was at Mt. Sinai that he began to develop the leadership skills that he would later display in running his own lab and dealing with bureaucracy.

From the beginning the situation at Mt. Sinai was tense because the hospital paid its interns and resident doctors poorly. Salk was elected president of the house staff, a position that required him to act as an intermediary between the staff and the administration of the hospital. Despite the weight of this added responsibility, Salk received the highest evaluations of any intern for his work with patients in his first year and was made responsible for advising new interns and instructing them in their duties in his second year. He inspired admiration and trust in everyone he worked with and treated.

The two years Salk was at Mt. Sinai were a very tumultuous time in the world. The United States was on the verge of plunging into World War II. Many of the doctors and interns showed their support for the war effort by wearing patriotic badges on their uniforms. When the bureaucrats who ran the hospital saw the badges, they immediately called Salk, the staff representative, and told him the badges had to disappear immediately because they were not permitted by hospital regulations.

Salk had a personal interest in the war—his brother Lee was in the army—and he knew that other people on the staff also had a strong sense of personal involvement in the war effort. Wearing the badges was very good for their morale; it made them feel they were doing more to support their friends,

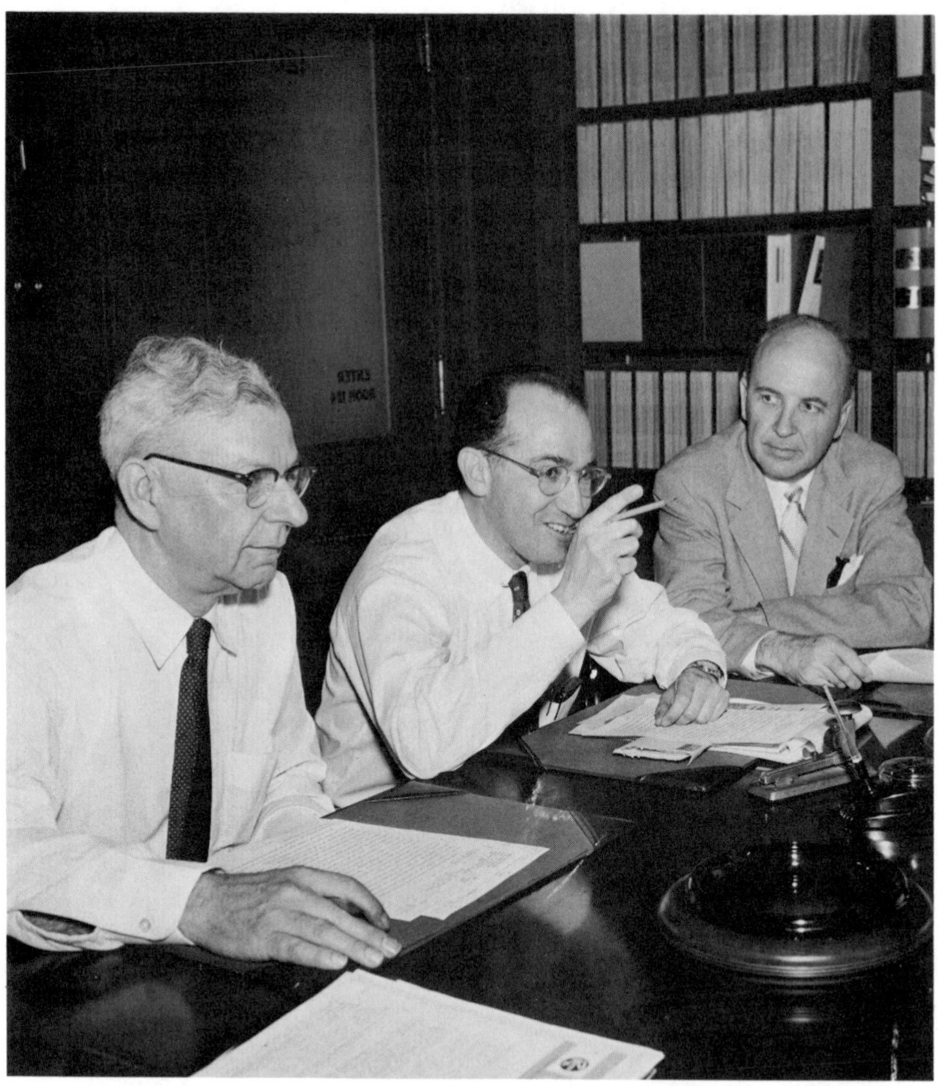

*At the National Institutes of Health in Washington, D.C., Salk meets with other members of a polio vaccine panel, in 1955: (from left) Secretary of the National Institute of Health Dr. William Workman, Dr. Jonas Salk, and Director of the National Institute of Health Dr. W. H. Sebrell, Jr.* (AP/Wide World Photos)

family, and country in hard times. Salk told the staff of the administration's order, and when they voted to continue wearing the badges he steadfastly represented them. The hospital threatened to deny any staff members wearing badges appointments to better jobs, but Salk knew he had the staff behind him and refused to budge. Throughout the negotiations, he maintained a calm perseverance. Eventually the administration was forced to back off and allow the staff to wear the badges.

## Influenza Work

In 1942, Salk finished his internship. His ambition was to pursue his research in virology. He had a very strong résumé of research experience and the highest recommendations from everyone he had worked with in medical school, but something he had no control over slowed him at first. Salk applied to many research institutes in New York but was turned down by all of them because he was Jewish. Anti-Semitic feelings were very strong in the medical community at that time.

Salk was extremely upset, but he did not allow anti-Semitism to discourage him. His mentor, Dr. Francis, was now the head of department of epidemiology at the University of Michigan, and Salk wrote to him for help and advice. Francis was surprised to find Salk available and moved to take advantage of his good fortune. He scraped together as much money as he could and offered Salk a job as an assistant in his influenza studies for forty dollars a week. Although his family and his young bride would have preferred that he stay in New York, Salk jumped at the opportunity to join Francis in Michigan.

During the war, influenza was a big threat to soldiers who lived in cramped barracks where disease was easily spread. The influenza work Francis was doing was well funded by the army and given urgent priority. As one of Francis' top assistants, Salk had the opportunity to learn the practical skills needed to run large experiments under pressure of time. When he wasn't traveling, he was able to learn the delicate lab techniques that he would later use in conquering polio.

The influenza vaccine that Salk helped Francis develop saved thousands of lives. What they did was also very much against the orthodoxy of viral studies; they killed viruses to make a vaccine. It was difficult and often tedious work. There are actually many different viruses, called strains, that cause influenza. All the strains of the influenza virus cause the same disease, but they can be different from one another in structure, size, and many other ways. In making a vaccine, the goal is to identify the properties and propensities of all strains of a virus, so that the vaccine will provide total immunity.

To make an influenza vaccine, Francis first had to isolate the influenza virus strains that caused infections—there were more than one hundred, and to miss any would make the vaccine less effective—before he could kill them in a test tube. He then had to try various formulas of the vaccine to see if the vaccine stimulated the immune system. This process took several years.

In 1943, Francis—with Salk as his assistant—was ready to test the influenza vaccine. Thousands of soldiers participated in the test: Some were injected with the vaccine and some with a placebo to find out if the vaccine actually worked. The number of soldiers who got influenza when injected with the placebo versus the number who got it when injected with the real vaccine would tell how well the vaccine worked.

Salk traveled all over the United States and Europe organizing and supervising trials once a vaccine was made. In the summer of 1944, the results were available: 70 percent fewer cases of influenza were reported among soldiers who had received the real vaccine.

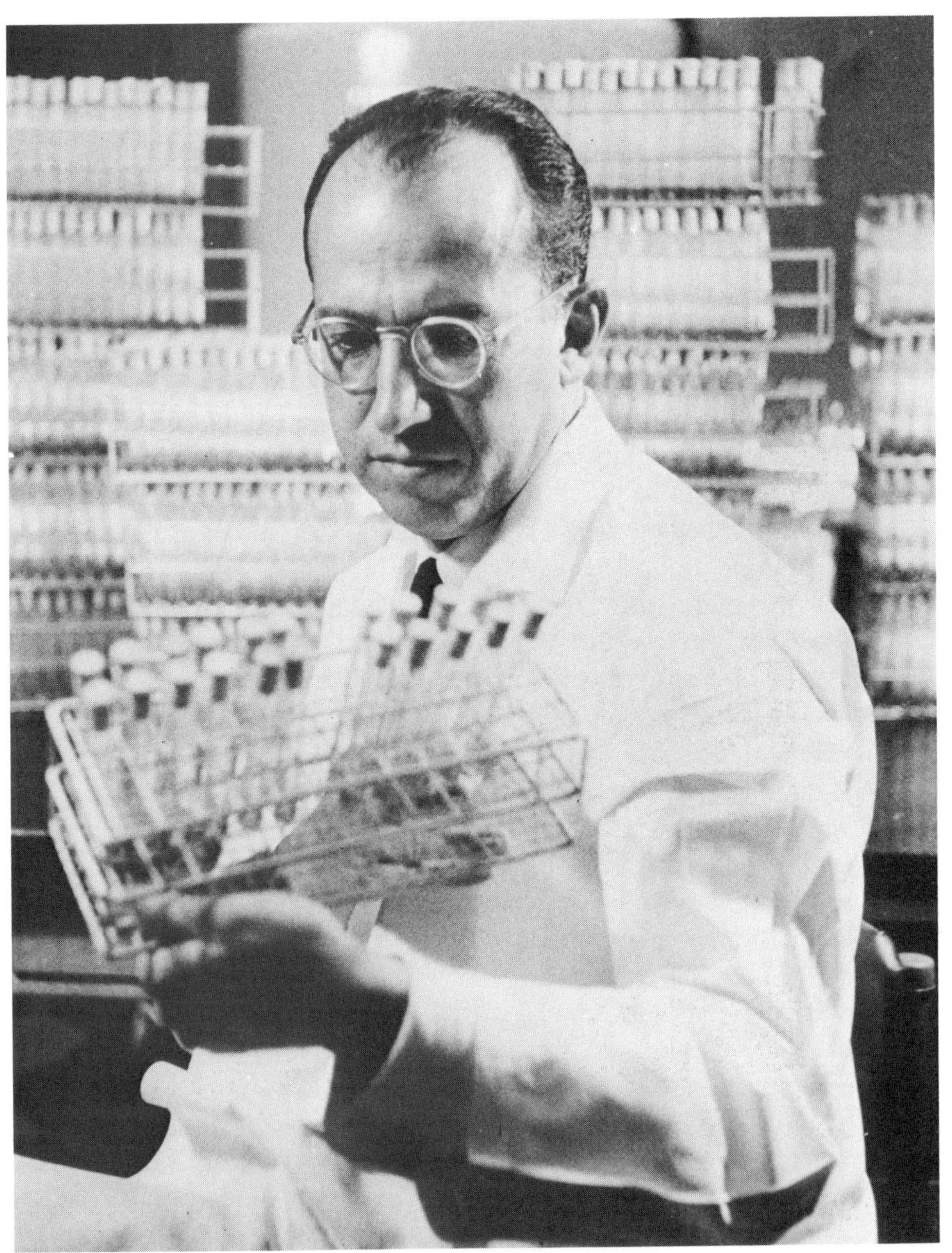

*Salk in his laboratory in 1954.* (AP/Wide World Photos)

## A Lab of His Own

After the war Salk began to become less and less comfortable working for Francis. Salk still respected and admired Francis; the trouble was that Francis designed and organized all the experiments. Salk felt that he was ready to direct his own laboratory. He began searching for a place where he could run his own show. This search led him to the University of Pittsburgh, where, in 1947, he accepted the position of resident virologist.

It was not an ideal situation for Salk. Were it not for his great resourcefulness, he most likely would have returned to work as an assistant for Francis or another virologist. When Salk arrived to begin his new job, he found he was to be housed in the basement of the Municipal Hospital of Pittsburgh. The rooms were small and full of excess furniture that was being stored there. Salk would have to renovate the space for it to function as a lab. Additionally, at that time Pittsburgh was a very polluted city because of all the coal-burning steel factories; every square inch of Salk's potential lab space was covered with fine black dust.

Salk quickly learned that the process of outfitting his lab was going to require single-minded determination and single-handed effort. Since his position was a new one, he fell between the cracks of the university bureaucracy, and no one seemed to know what to do with him. The building was owned by the city, Salk's operating budget came from the university's physics department, and he was a faculty member of the medical school. Every step he took, from building a test-tube agitating rack to buying paper clips, required the approval of all the different departments. Salk found that much of his time was taken up signing triplicates of requisitions for the materials and money he needed.

Salk's ambition had been to have his own lab and to do his own research. Now that he had his lab, however, he had a whole new set of problems to take on—problems which had nothing to do with medical research that would give people healthier lives. Salk had always believed that if the deck was stacked against him he would simply work twice as hard as he had before and his hard work would prevail. In 1947, he discovered that even though he was a respected researcher, he was not assured of being able to do the work he knew was valuable and needed in the world. After a couple of months in Pittsburgh, Salk began to wonder if he had made a mistake in setting out on his own.

# Chapter 4

# The Polio Vaccine

Five years later, Salk was still in Pittsburgh, but his circumstances had changed a great deal. Sometime early in 1952, Dr. Salk filled a syringe with a pink liquid, held it to the light to be sure he had the proper measurement, and then injected the liquid into his arm. He was the first human being to receive the polio vaccine that he and his lab staff had created.

Salk knew that he was taking a risk when he inoculated himself. Inoculating himself would make it harder for him to remain detached about tests on the vaccine. His health would be at stake in every test result. Numerous lab animals had received the vaccine and had not developed polio, but this was no guarantee that the reaction would not be different in humans. It would be two years before extensive tests on hundreds of thousands of people would prove that the vaccine Salk synthesized was safe and effective in preventing polio.

In 1952, however, Salk was so confident that his vaccine would work that he made sure he was the first person to receive it and test its effectiveness and safety. Shortly thereafter, his entire lab staff would be vaccinated. Then, in the ultimate sign of his confidence in his creation, Salk inoculated his three sons and his wife. (His compassion was always evident; he vaccinated his children while they slept, so they would not be frightened by the needles.)

In May, 1952, after five months of haggling, Salk was given official clearance to begin testing his vaccine on patients at the Polk State School for retarded welfare recipients and the D.T. Watson Home for Crippled Children. He performed all these inoculations personally. During these first tests, Salk was around the Watson Home so often, checking to make sure the children were OK, that the cook was able to find out what his favorite kind of pie was—strawberry—and bake it whenever he was there.

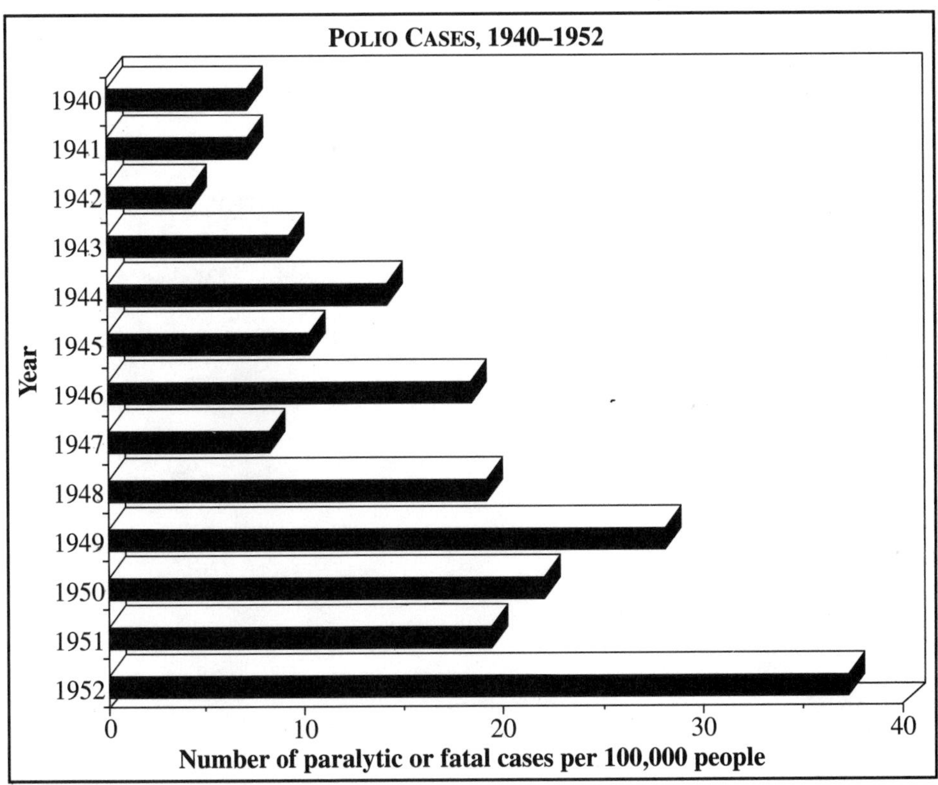


## Helping Hands

In the process of getting to the point of publicly testing the vaccine, Salk's basement lab had expanded to occupy the three floors above him. This same growing lab now had twenty-five full-time employees. Salk's responsibilities were staggering.

Between running the experiments and administering the lab, he routinely worked sixteen-hour days. The lab was receiving up to a thousand white mice a week, hundreds of chickens, hundreds of ground squirrels, and at least fifty monkeys a week as well. The research required ten thousand test tubes a month and countless other lab materials, from white lab coats to centrifuges and microscopes.

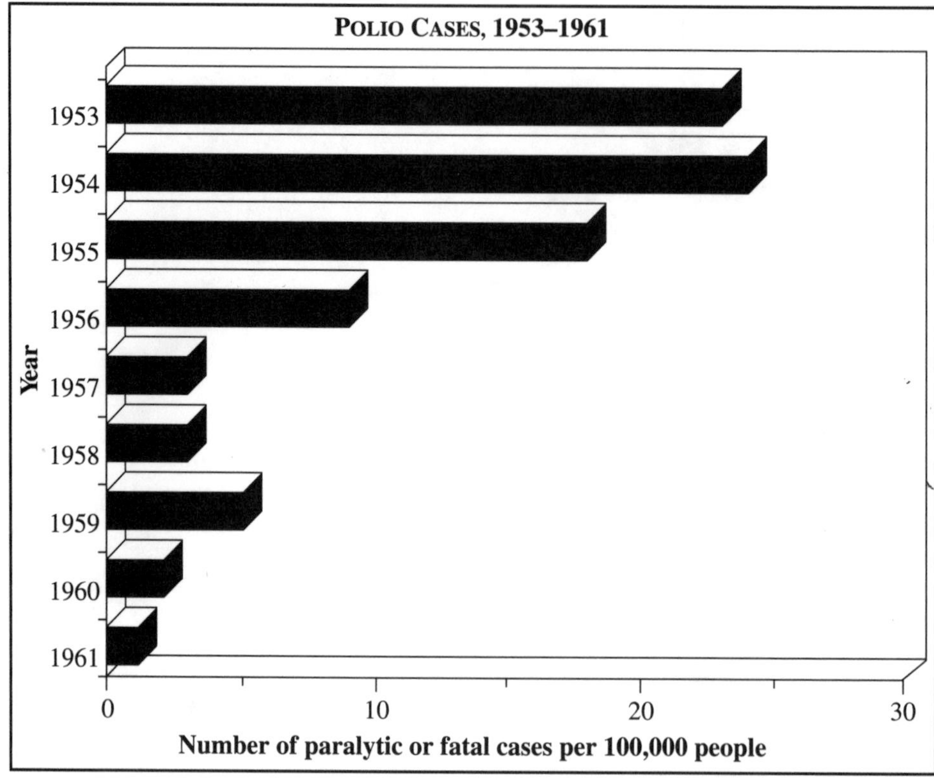


At last, as he had long hoped, Salk was designing his own experiments. The development of the lab was a tribute to his creativity, his organizational skills, and his capacity for head-splitting, hard work. Still, the creation of the polio vaccine wasn't accomplished solely by Salk. In particular, Salk was helped by the National Foundation for Infantile Paralysis, better known as the March of Dimes, which drew him to the study of polio and funded his research, and by the work of another scientist, John Enders, who found a way to grow the polio virus in tissue cultures, outside a living body.

The March of Dimes had been supporting research on polio since the 1920's, when Franklin Delano Roosevelt—soon to become president of the United States—contracted the disease and became paralyzed below the waist. Roosevelt founded the March of Dimes to help poorer paralysis victims pay for the expensive braces and rehabilitation that were needed after the disease had run its course. In time, as epidemics continued to ravage the country, the March of Dimes made vanquishing polio completely through vaccine research one of its main goals.

By 1947, the scientists whose research the March of Dimes had supported had determined that it was necessary to find out how many types of polio virus there were before a vaccine could be made that would stop the disease. Since each strain of a polio virus acts differently from other strains, an effective vaccine would have to contain all strains of polio.

The process of identifying all strains of a virus was a very time-consuming activity. For the most part, the established virologists of the day preferred to let others perform this essential but highly tedious work. As a result, younger, hungrier researchers were contracted to do it.

In 1947, Salk was bogged down in his work on influenza. He lacked the space and the funding that would allow him to carry out more effective experiments. Fortunately, the work he had done with Dr. Francis had built him a good reputation. On that basis, Salk was recommended to the March of Dimes as a bright young researcher who might be interested in working on

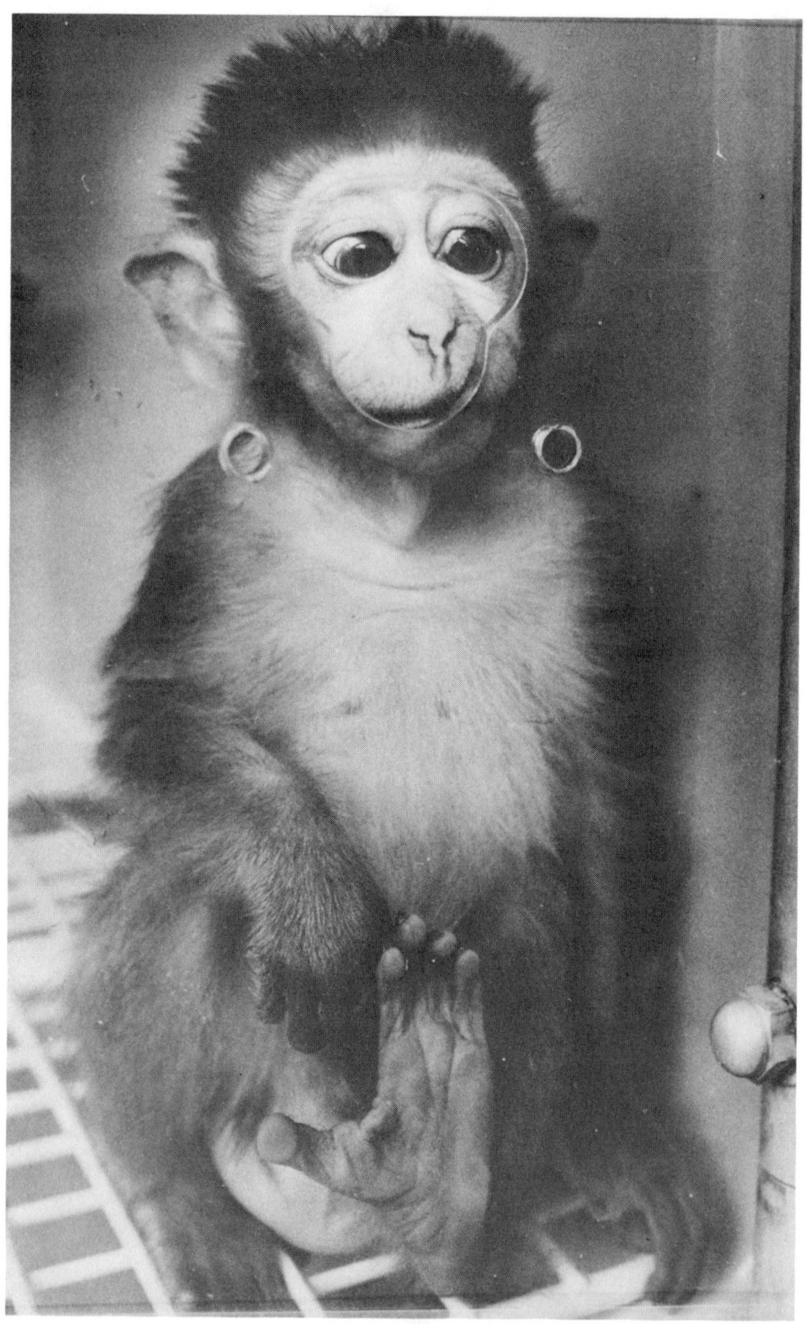

*Monkeys played a vital role in Salk's research to develop the polio vaccine.*
(AP/Wide World Photos)

the polio virus-typing program. Even though Salk had never worked with polio before, he quickly accepted the offer to join the typing project because he knew it would allow him to build a well-equipped lab and do research that would have immediate and life-saving implications. Salk knew the work would be slow, but he figured he would be able to find a way to speed it up and make it more bearable.

**Monkeys and Polio Research**

*Rhesus monkeys were the unsung heroes of polio research; no vaccines could have been made without them. They are the only animals which polio will infect naturally. Trappers caught them in the jungles of India and the Philippines, and then they were flown to New York on special planes with a full-time flight attendant to feed and care for them. Okatie Farms, in South Carolina, held the monkeys for three weeks to make sure they were healthy and then transported them to the labs.*

*In the labs the monkeys were injected with polio virus and test vaccines or killed and their kidneys minced to grow polio virus. In 1955, more than five thousand monkeys were used each month for polio research. Each monkey yielded about 850 doses of Salk vaccine. Today fewer monkeys are used in research, in part as a result of advances in lab techniques and in part in response to the protests of animal rights activists.*

The opportunity to speed things along was provided by Dr. Enders. In 1948 and 1949, while Salk's lab was being outfitted and he was starting the typing program, Enders was working on growing chicken-pox viruses in bits of human embryo tissue kept alive in test tubes. At the end of an experiment, he had a few test tubes left and decided to put some polio viruses into the test tubes to see what would happen. Conventional wisdom said that polio grew only in nervous tissues, so Enders was surprised to find that the polio virus had grown in the cultures when he tested them later. He announced his discovery at a meeting of virologists in 1949; Salk was one of the first to understand and apply the techniques Enders had discovered.

Enders' work (for which he and two other researchers received a Nobel Prize in 1954) was significant not only for polio research but also for virology in general. It allowed scientists to isolate and propagate different strains of the viruses they were studying with much greater efficiency.

In practical terms, Enders' discovery saved monkeys and saved time. Monkeys are the only organisms besides humans who can become infected by the polio virus and develop polio. The various scientists doing polio research used thousands of monkeys (see sidebar) in the course of their studies. Furthermore, the only way to obtain the polio virus was from a person or monkey who was infected. Before Enders' discovery, the only way to run tests on the virus was to infect a body with it. Since no researcher would dream of infecting a human being with a deadly virus, monkeys were the test subjects.

The typing program that Salk was working on called for him to give a dose of a *known* strain of polio virus to a monkey and let the disease run its course. If the monkey's immune system developed antibodies for that strain of polio and the monkey recovered, Salk was to give the monkey a shot of an *unclassified* type of polio virus and see if it got sick. If the monkey got sick again, then the second strain of polio virus was different from the first (the monkey did not have antibodies for it) and the whole process was run again. If the monkey didn't get sick, the second—previously unclassified—virus could be classified as the same type as the first.

This testing process was frustratingly inefficient. Monkeys took months to recover from each infection. When they died, more time was lost. Because of this, the original experiment was to run for more than three years. When Salk rearranged the experiment using tissue cultures instead of live monkeys, he was able to complete the typing in a matter of months. The tissue cultures provided a stage for the cellular activity of a virus attacking an organism without all the maintenance that an entire organism required. Not only that, tissue cultures were much more economical than monkeys.

Salk did not stop with improving the typing program, he took the ball and ran with it. Applying the ideas of inactivating viruses with formalin he had learned by working with influenza, he realized that once the types of polio had been identified, he could make a dead-virus vaccine for polio just as he and Francis had with influenza. The leading virologists said that a dead-cell vaccine would not work with polio, but Salk saw no reason why it shouldn't and less reason why it should not be tried.

In 1951, Jonas Salk announced to the International Conference on Poliomyelitis in Denmark that his work in the typing program had determined that there were three types of polio virus (called Mahoney, Saukett, and Lansing after the people they were taken from). It was his first major independent research accomplishment. On the ship back to America, Salk spent a great deal of time talking with Basil O'Connor, the fiery, down-to-earth, and controversial figure who had led the March of Dimes from its inception.

In the course of the cruise, O'Connor and Salk discovered they had a great deal in common. Both men came from impoverished, immigrant backgrounds and had risen to positions of respect through hard work and an ability to see things in a larger context. In addition, both were impatient with orthodoxy.

O'Connor's organization had been battling against polio for decades. Here suddenly was a researcher confident that he could develop an effective polio vaccine within a couple of years. By the end of the cruise, O'Connor had promised that the March of Dimes would provide the support Salk needed to develop and test his vaccine.

## Battling the Medical Establishment

Although the support of the March of Dimes was a boon for Salk's lab building and experiment financing, it did not make him many friends among his fellow scientists. Many of the world's most renowned virologists did not think the line of research Salk was pursuing was the best way to eliminate polio. They believed that a live-virus vaccine would work better. They said it would take at least twenty years to test a killed-virus vaccine to make sure it was safe.

The majority of other scientists felt it was a waste of money to work on killed-virus research when so many experts were sure it would fail. These scientists said there was no way to be sure you had killed all the viruses and still cause an immune response. They feared that an improperly made killed-virus vaccine would contain some live, virulent virus and thus would cause the disease it was meant to prevent. Many of these same scientists also felt that Salk was "selling out" to the March of Dimes by accepting such large amounts of money to fund his research. They feared he would feel compelled to deliver results to the March of Dimes's liking and thus would compromise his scientific integrity and objectivity.

Salk, however, was extremely confident of his methods and intentions and saw the March of Dimes's money only as a facilitator for his very practical and timely experiments. In the early 1950's, the number of polio cases reported was increasing dramatically every year. Salk saw the need to work quickly and forgo convention so that fewer people would suffer from polio. That Salk stuck to his convictions and did not bow to the opinions of the "leading" minds in his field was to make him enemies who would dog him and his vaccine for the rest of his career.

## Passing the Test

Salk did work quickly. After testing his vaccine on humans on a small scale in 1952, he worked through the resistance of his peers and planned a test that would allow him to find out if his vaccine was safe and effective in one year rather than twenty. By 1954, Salk was ready for a large-scale test. With

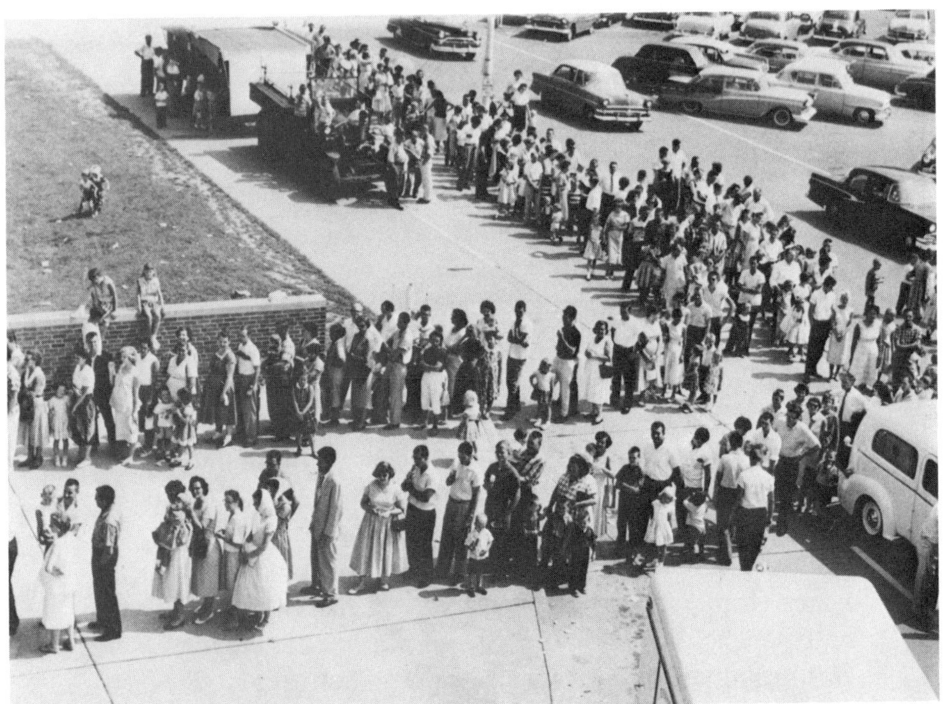

*On this day in 1959 at the Municipal Stadium in Evansville, Indiana, some fourteen thousand people were inoculated with the Salk vaccine.* (AP/Wide World Photos)

the help of the March of Dimes and his old mentor, Dr. Francis, he designed one of the largest human trials ever attempted. More than 650,000 children in forty-four states received vaccine and more than a million other children were observed as a control group. Children were used because they were less likely to have developed antibodies naturally.

The great experiment began one morning in April, 1954, when first through third graders all across the country poured out of class and lined up in the gym or school auditorium to receive the vaccine. In the South, where black and white children were still forced to go to separate schools, the black children were marched to the white schools for their inoculations but had to wait on the lawn because they were not allowed in the same building as the white kids. In California, the weather was hot, and the faces of the nervous children were beaded with sweat. In the Northeast, kids in cities and kids in the country lined up for their vaccines.

At all of the hundreds of inoculation sites, the nurses and doctors running the show quickly vaccinated the children and then rewarded them for their courage with a lollipop. Over the course of the summer, the test kids would receive booster shots or have blood samples taken to determine how much antibody the vaccine was causing the body to produce. At the end of the summer, the kids received a badge that said "Polio Pioneer," letting the world know that they had taken part in the monumental test. Of course, the real advantage gained for the polio pioneers was that they were vaccinated for polio.

Over the winter of 1954-1955, Dr. Francis collected the hundreds of pages of data that were generated from the test, and the whole world held its breath waiting for the test results. If it had turned out that the vaccine had not worked, Salk would have lost his credibility, the March of Dimes would have spent millions of dollars for nothing, and—most important—the public would have had to give up the hope of being free from the danger of polio for many years to come.

On April 12, 1955, Dr. Francis read the results to an audience of scientists and reporters, as well as to countless people watching on television and listening on radio. It was a media event unparalleled up to the time. The room was silent as the stern Francis rattled off figures from trials in each part of the country. The results showed that people who received the vaccine were 70 percent less likely to get polio than were people who had not been inoculated. Equally important, no one had contracted the disease from the vaccination itself. Salk's vaccine was both safe and effective.

The reporters at the scene ran to phones to rush this front-page story to newspapers around the world. Salk took the stage and promised he could make a vaccine that was even better than the one tested. By making this promise, Salk further angered his critics in the scientific community. Salk's intention was to express his determination to conquer polio completely. In the eyes of his critics, however, Salk was showboating, promising things that were still unproven. Salk's critics believed that he was raising the public's hopes recklessly, acting more like a circus promoter than a scientist.

The general public saw things differently. People were enormously relieved to learn that a vaccine against polio had been developed, and they were grateful to its creator. In their eyes, Salk was a hero. In the days following the announcement of the test results, Salk received so many thank-you calls that he had to have his phone disconnected. He received thousands of letters of thanks, and at first he tried to answer all of them personally. He was offered everything from cars to money as gifts and was contacted by numerous businesses that wanted him to endorse their products. Salk refused all the outpourings of material thanks and business offers. He was most interested in returning to the lab, but his celebrity would not allow this for many years to come.

## Tragedy

The public wanted to have Salk's vaccine as soon as

possible so that they could be protected from polio in the coming summer. Several pharmaceutical companies began making vaccine and selling it immediately after the test results were announced. In the rush to fill the public's demand, some batches of vaccine produced at Cutter Pharmaceutical in Berkeley, California, were made without sufficient care. As a result, live infectious viruses got into the vaccine. When this vaccine was injected into people, they got polio instead of being saved from it.

Two hundred and four people caught polio from the tainted vaccine before it was discovered and pulled off the market. Three quarters of these victims were paralyzed for life, and eleven died. Suddenly the public was not so sure of the vaccine. The scientists who had disagreed with Salk's methods and ideas poured out "I told you so's, " and the March of Dimes and the government scrambled to find out what had gone wrong. Salk was devastated by the thought that his vaccine had caused harm to anyone.

It was eventually discovered that mistakes made in the hurry to produce large amounts of vaccine were the cause of the tragedy, not the process Salk had developed. Still, the criticism from other scientists continued. One of Salk's main detractors, Dr. Albert Sabin, was particularly cutting in his criticism of Salk and the killed-virus vaccine. Sabin was convinced that an attenuated-virus vaccine would be more reliable, and the Cutter incident strengthened his determination to develop such a vaccine.

Salk was forced into a sort of hibernation in the summer of 1955. His fame baffled him and distracted him from his labwork. The alienation he felt from his fellow scientists also baffled him. The course of his life and thinking was to be unalterably changed by the fallout from his polio vaccine.

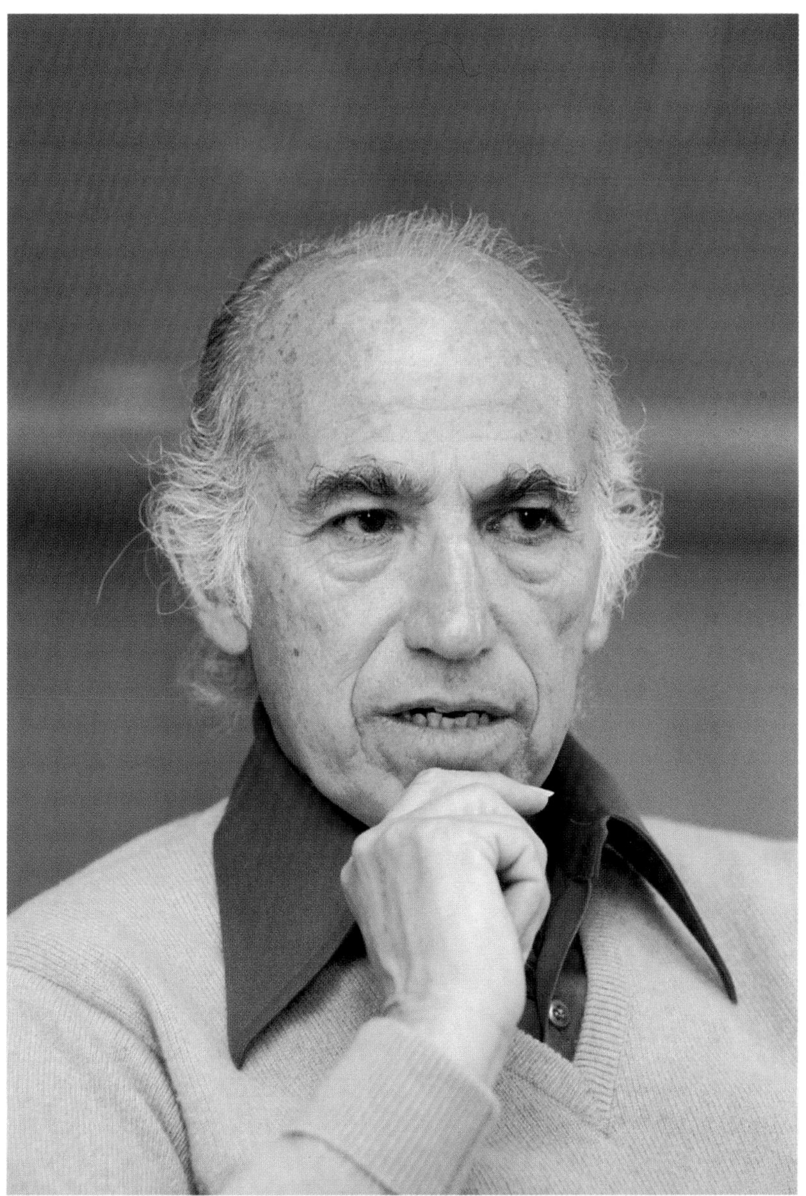

1. Jonas Salk. (AP/Wide World Photos)

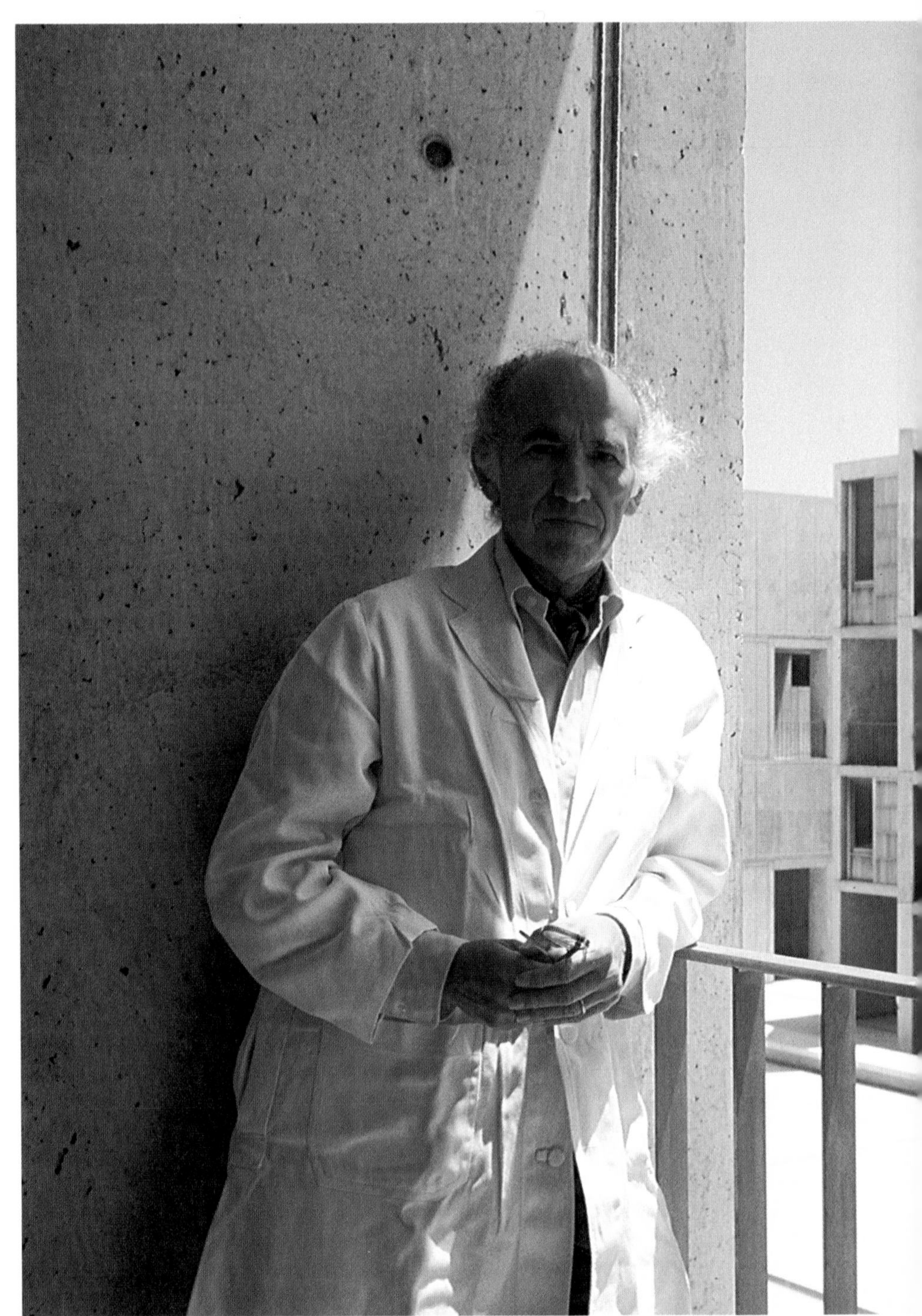

2. The Salk Institute. (Richard Gross Photo, Grants Pass, Oregon)

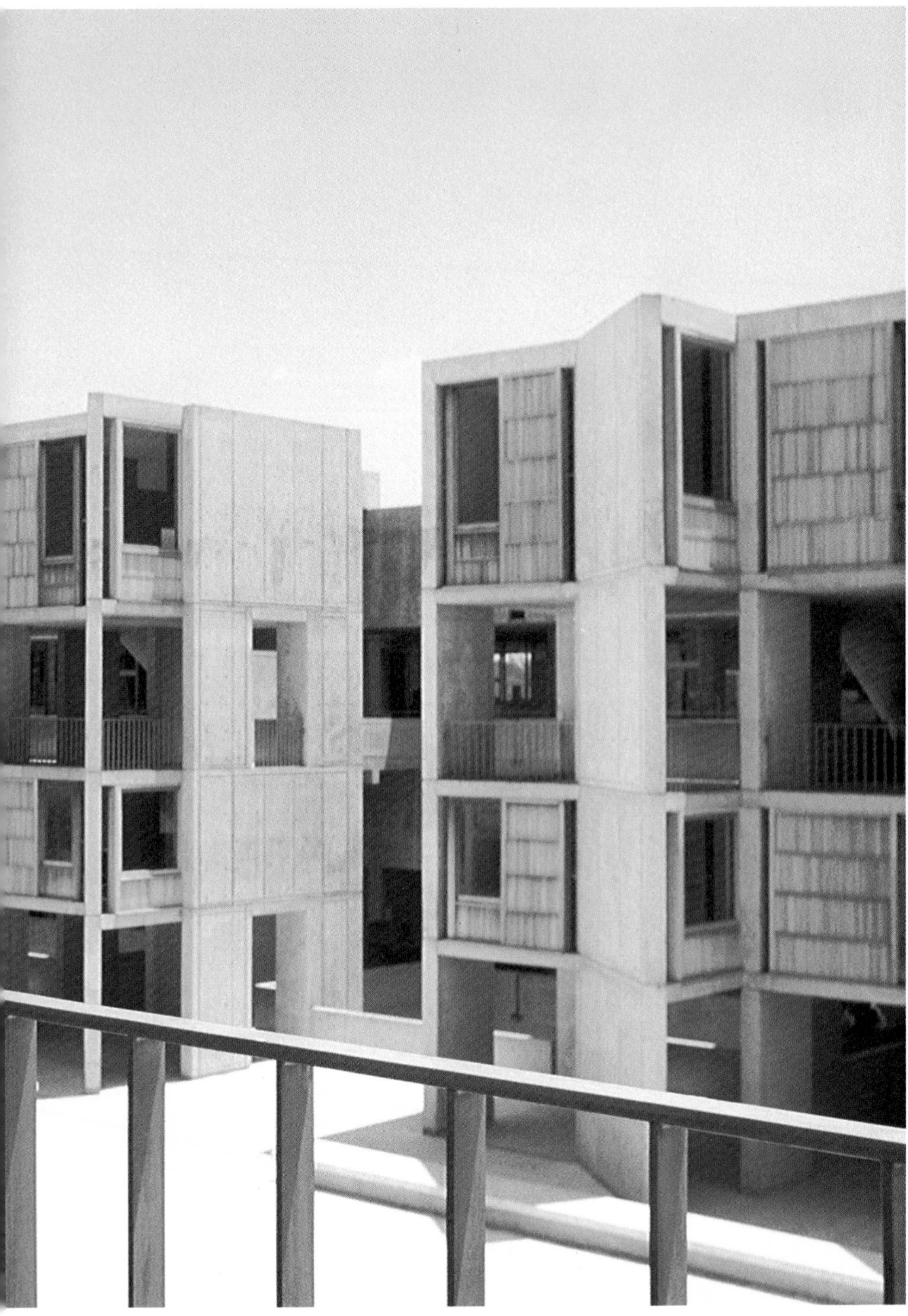

3. Salk with his wife, artist Françoise Gilot. (Richard Gross Photo, Grants Pass, Oregon)

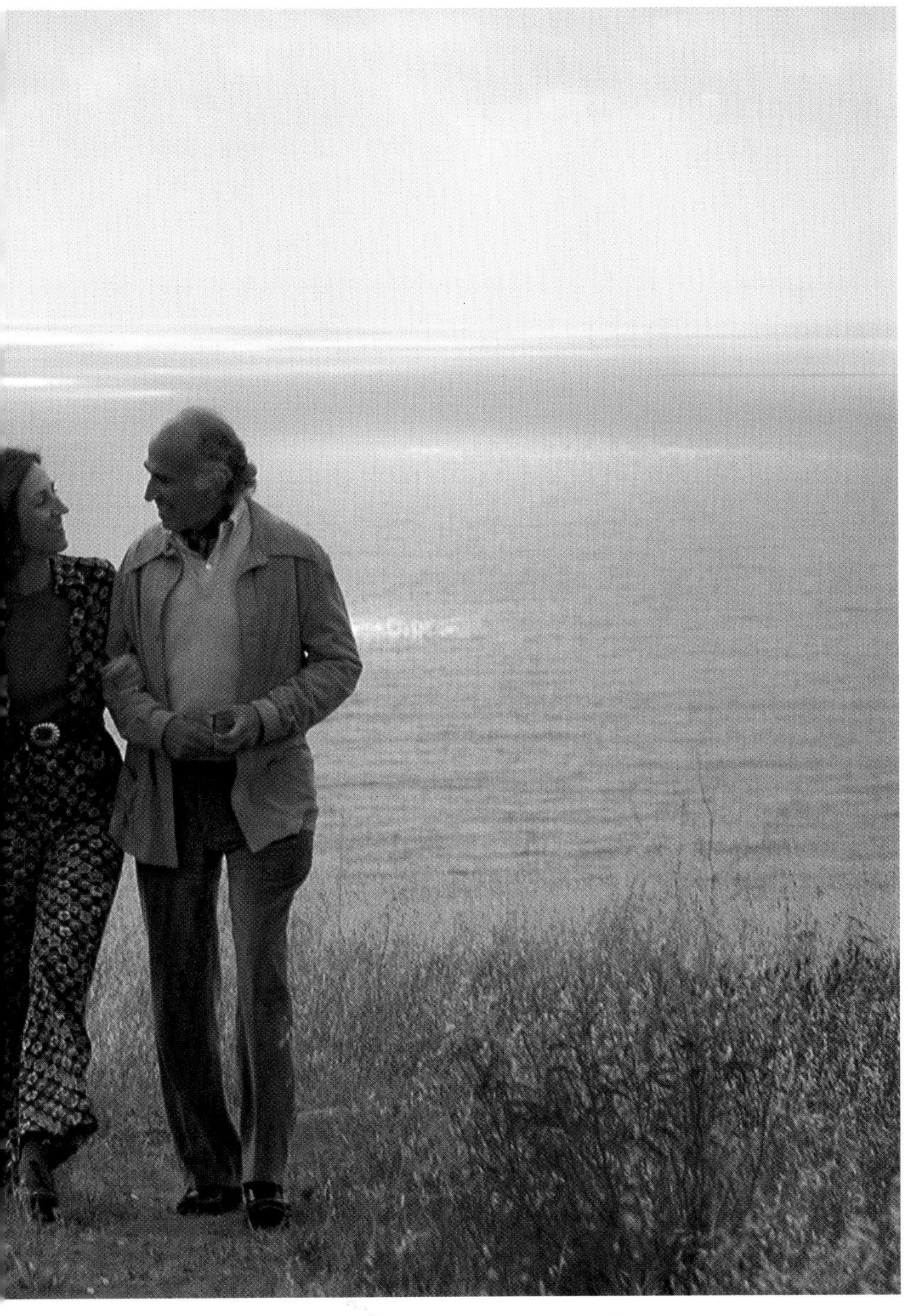

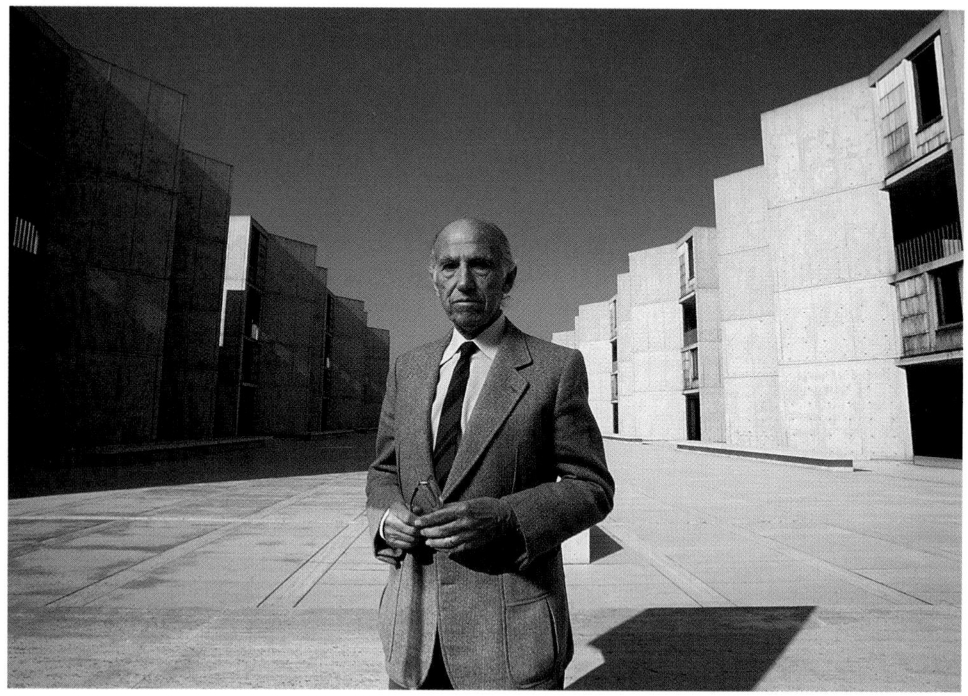

4. Salk's collaboration with architect Louis Kahn produced a masterpiece of modern design: The Salk Institute. (Karen Kasmauski/Woodfin Camp)

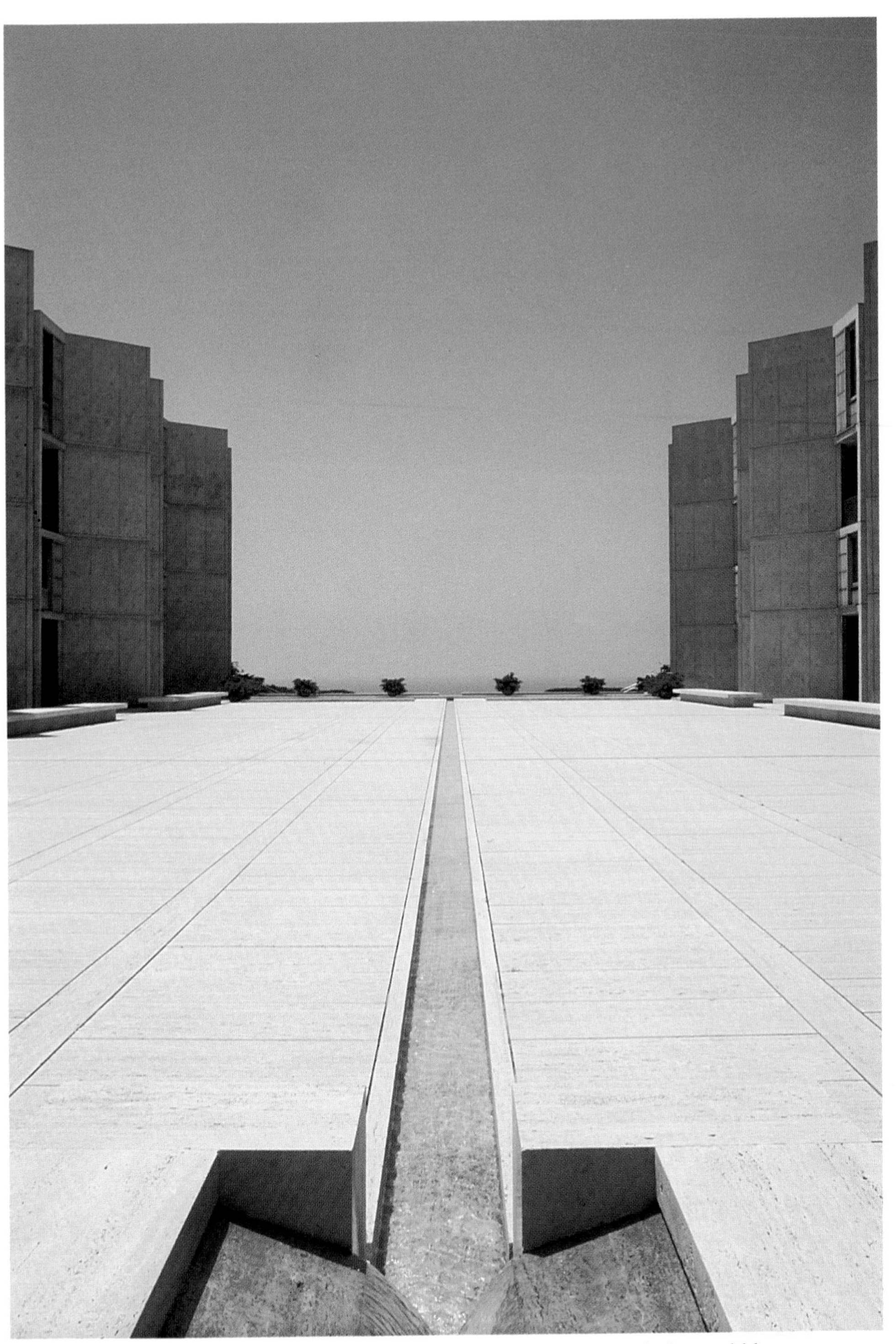

5. Salk envisioned the institute as a place where the world's great minds would learn from one another. (Richard Gross Photo, Grants Pass, Oregon)

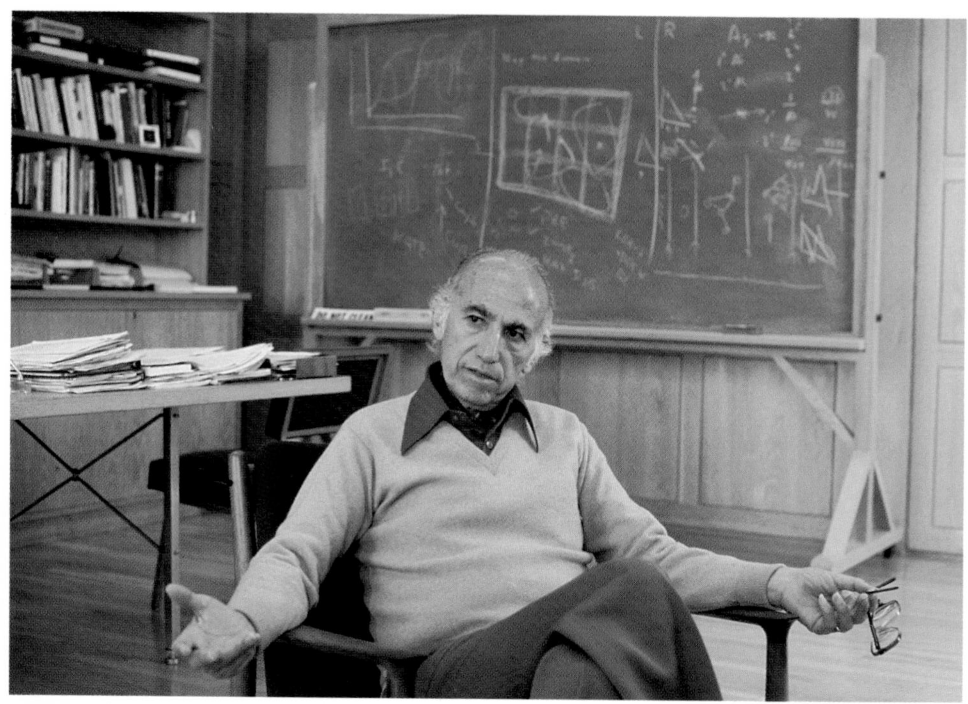

6. Salk's quest for understanding led him to develop a personal philosophy with an evolutionary perspective on humankind's place in the universe. (AP/Wide World Photos)

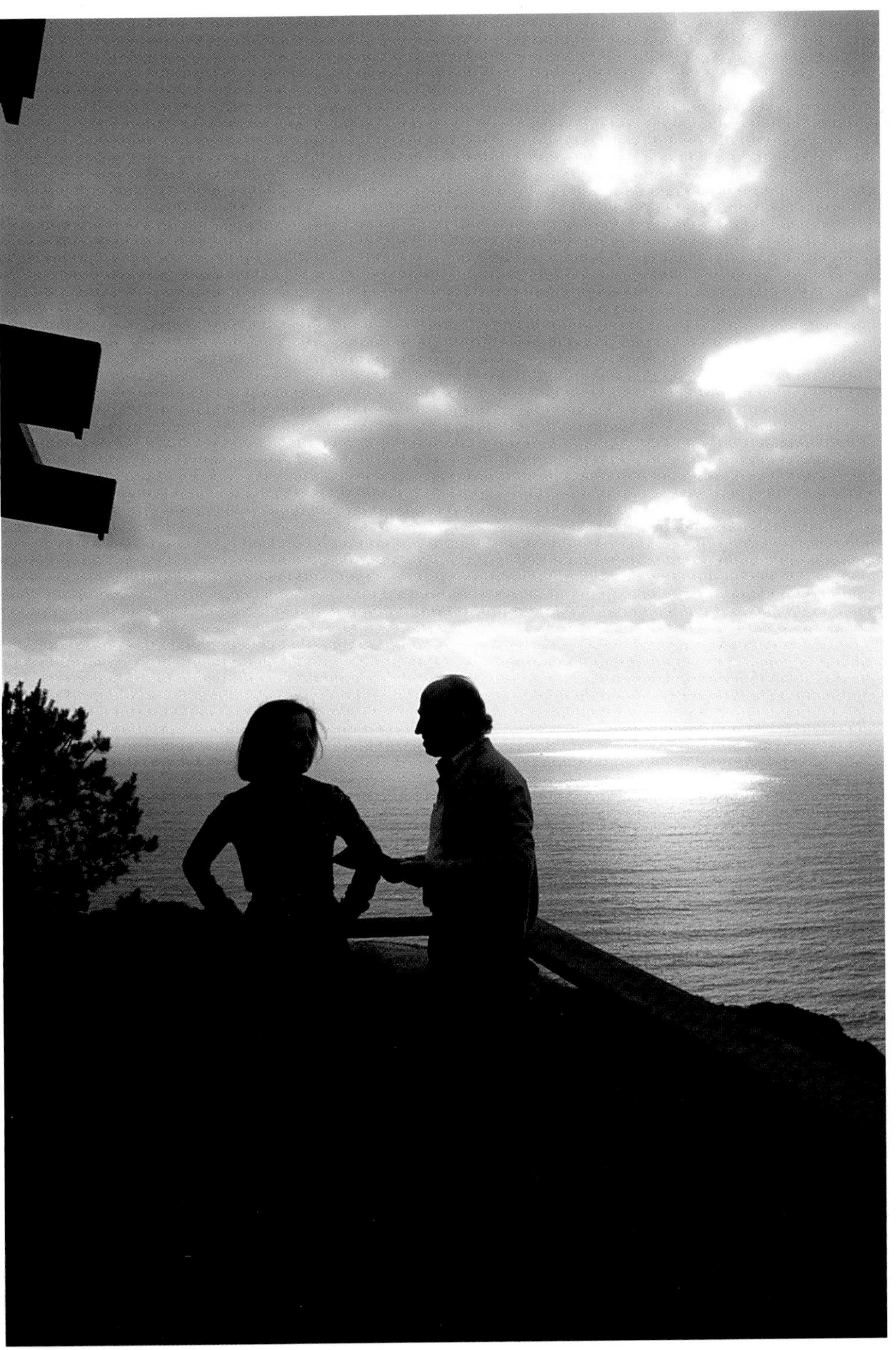

7. Gilot's artistic creativity was a stimulus to Salk's interdisciplinary research, which challenged conventional thinking. (Richard Gross Photo, Grants Pass, Oregon)

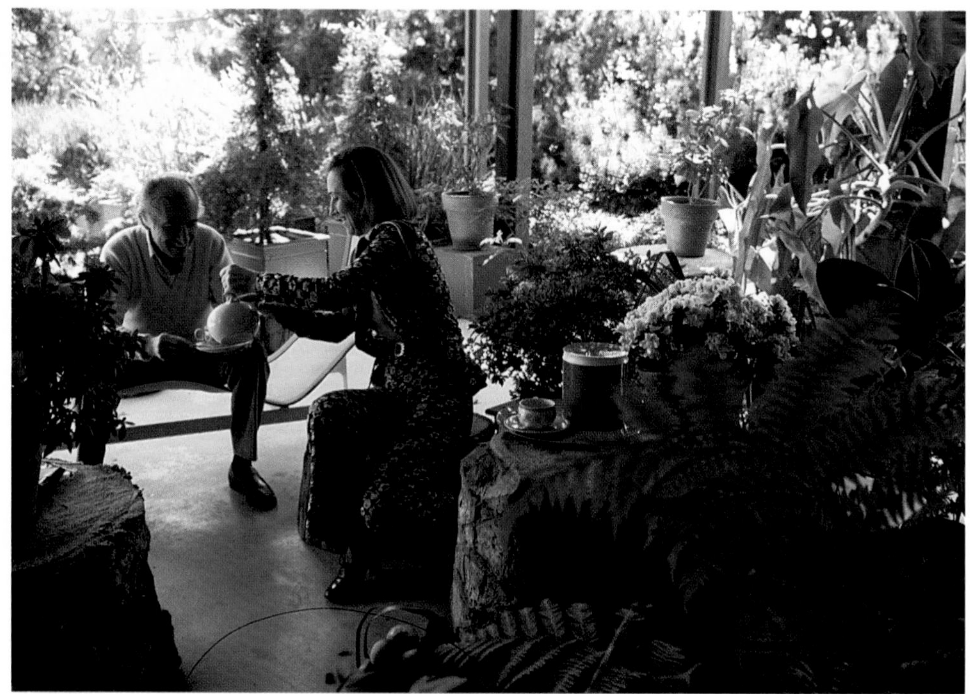

8. Two years after his marriage to Gilot, Salk published *Man Unfolding*, his first statement of his evolutionary philosophy. (Richard Gross Photo, Grants Pass, Oregon)

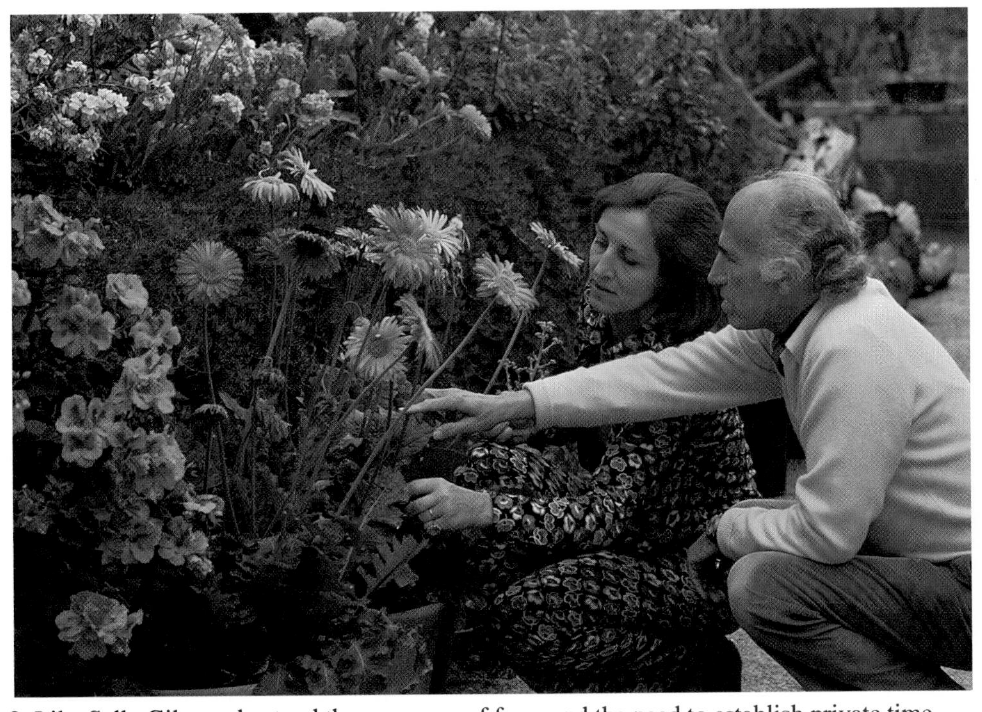

9. Like Salk, Gilot understood the pressures of fame and the need to establish private time.
(Richard Gross Photo, Grants Pass, Oregon)

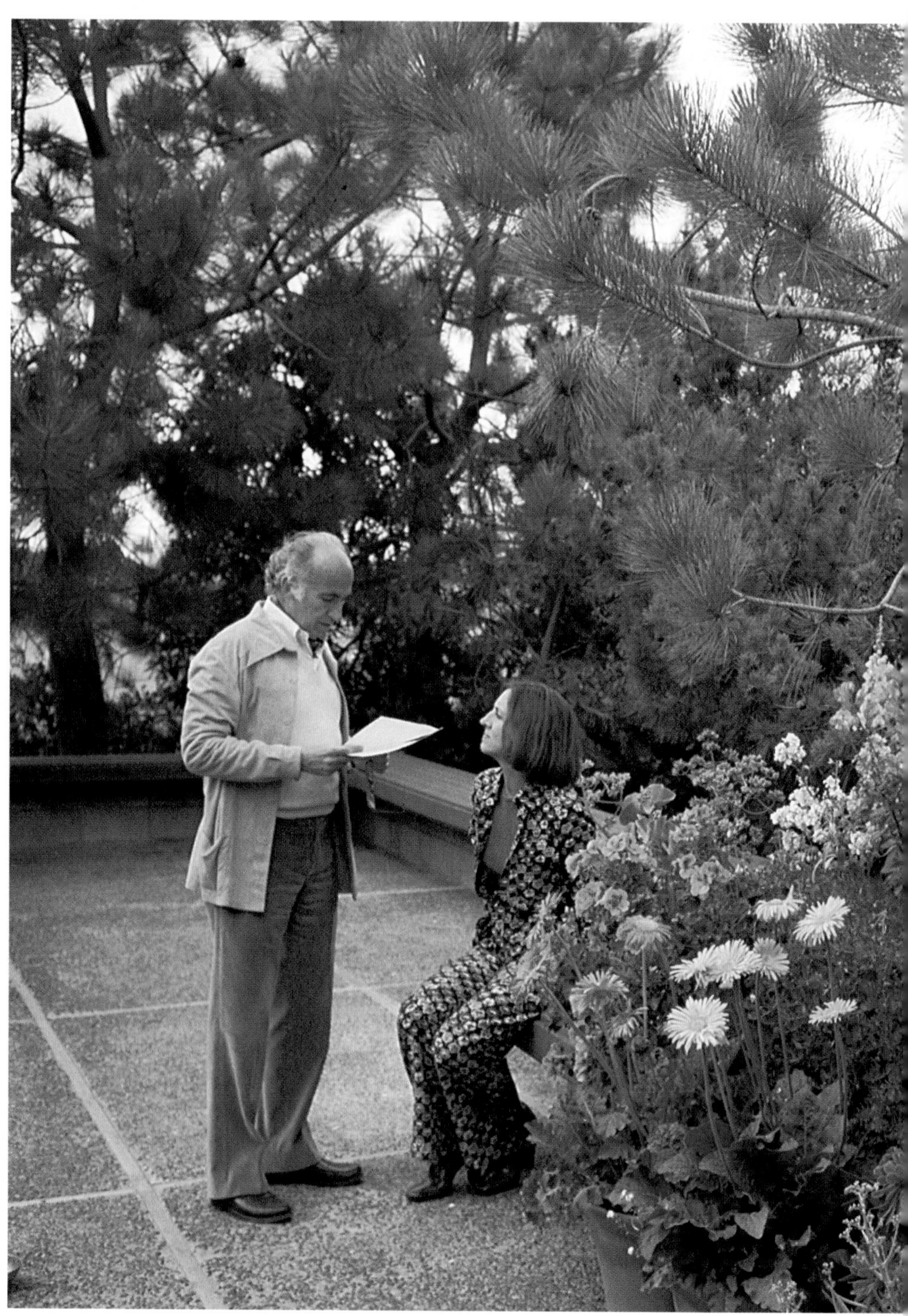

10. Artist and scientist, individual and society, mind and body: Salk believes that such polarities fuel evolutionary change. (Richard Gross Photo, Grants Pass, Oregon)

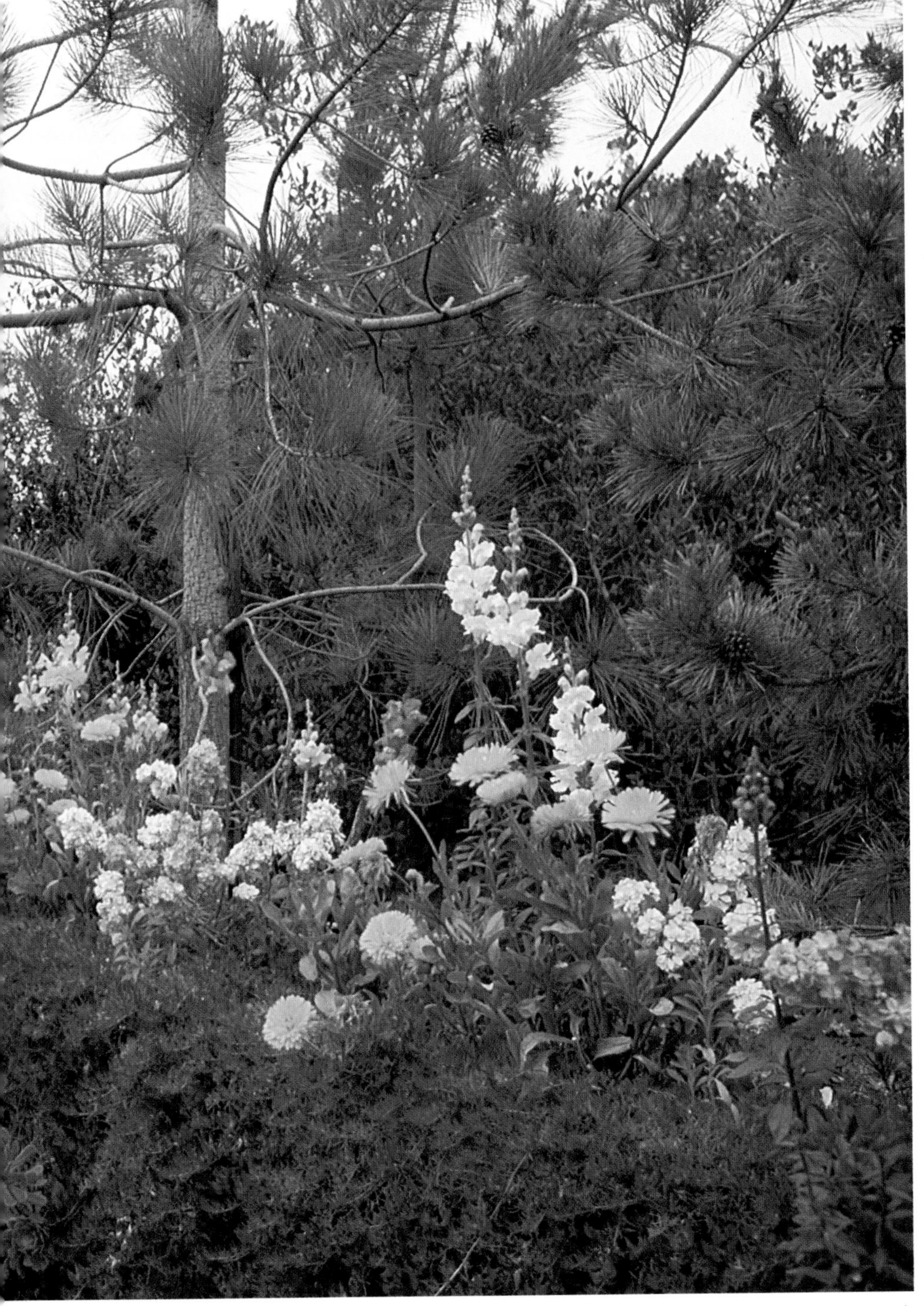

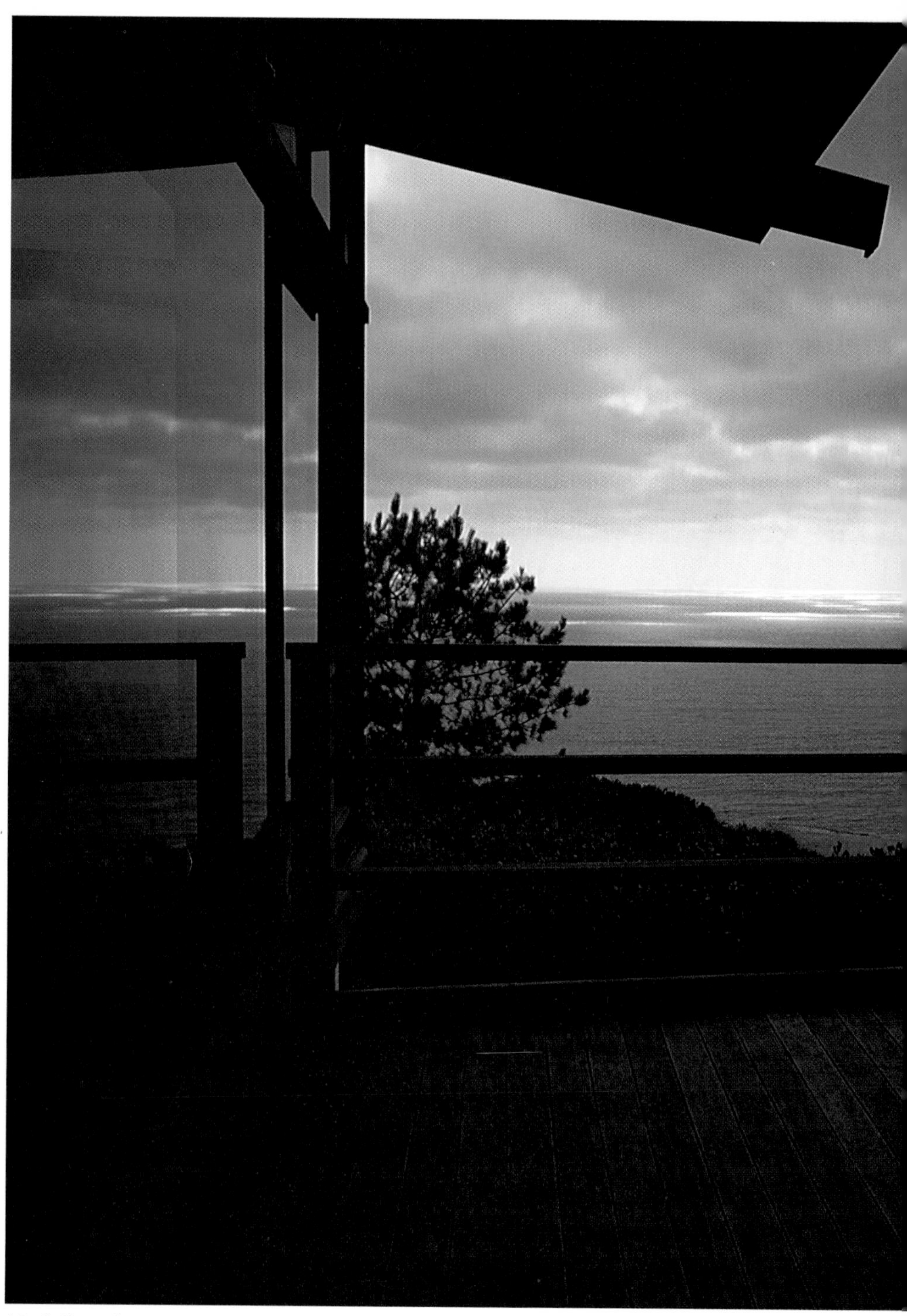

11. Salk at the tape recorder; often he wakes in the middle of the night to jot down or record new ideas. (Richard Gross Photo, Grants Pass, Oregon)

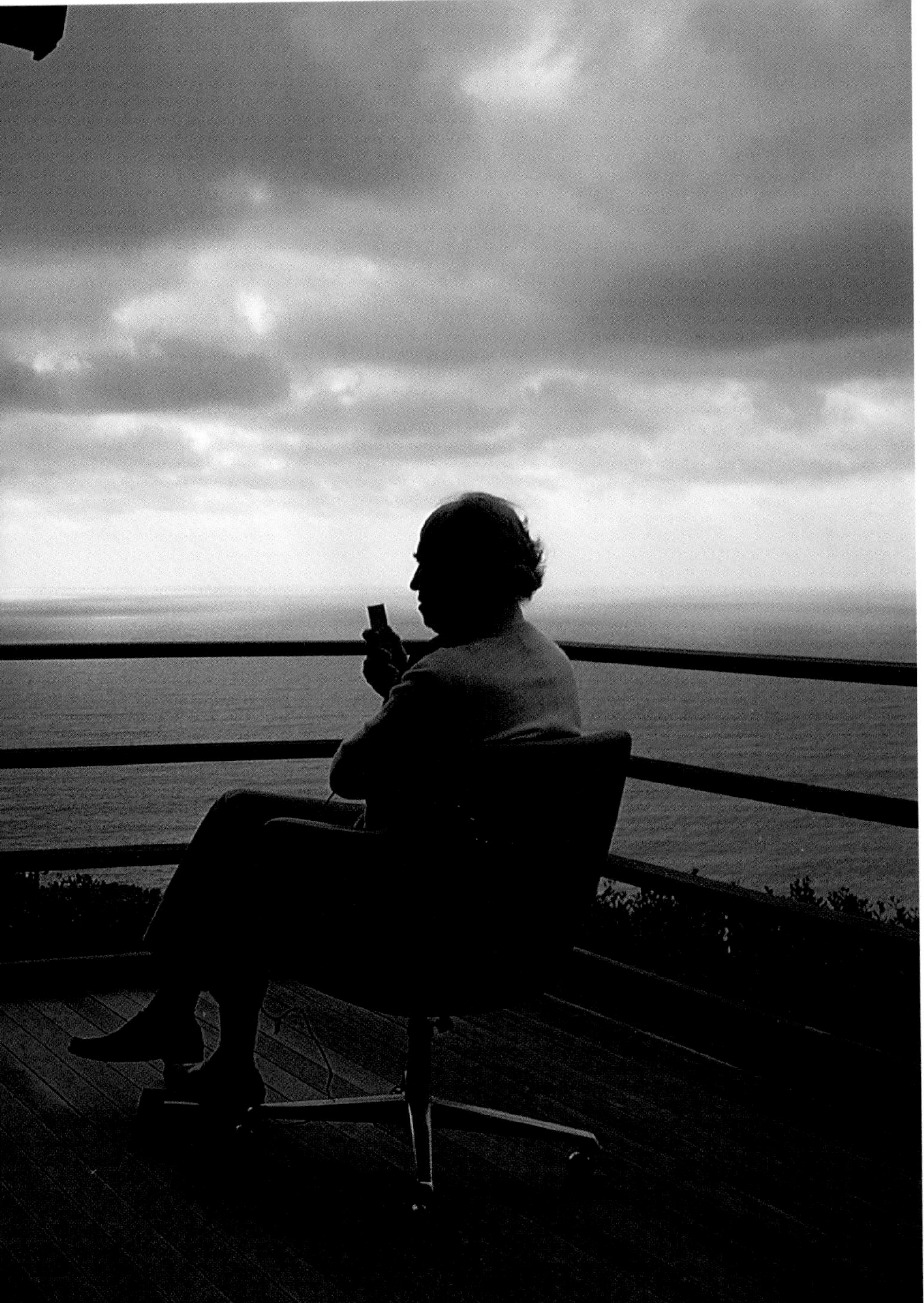

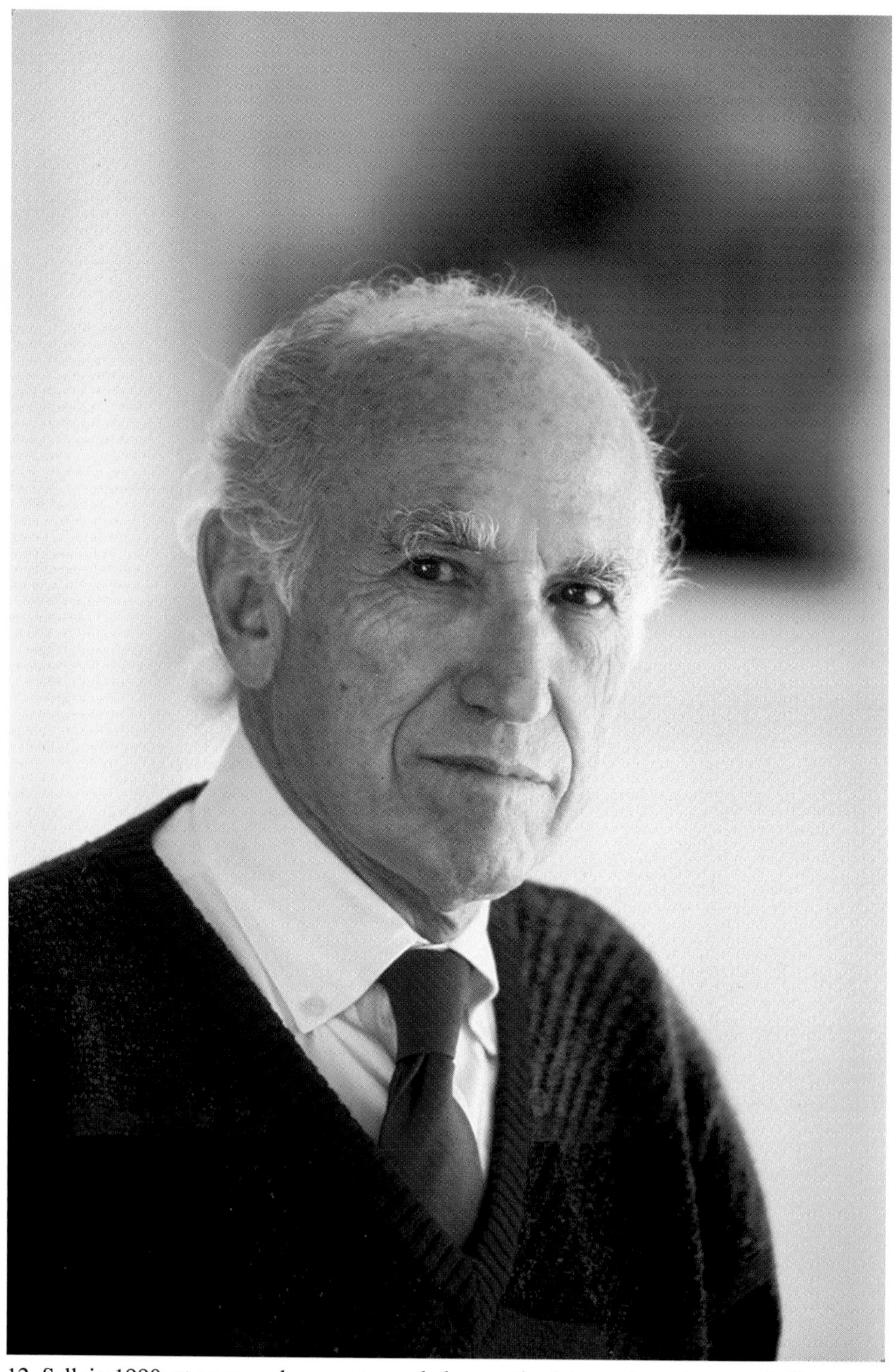

12. Salk in 1990; at an age when most people have retired, he took up the new challenge of AIDS research. (Lester Sloan/Woodfin Camp)

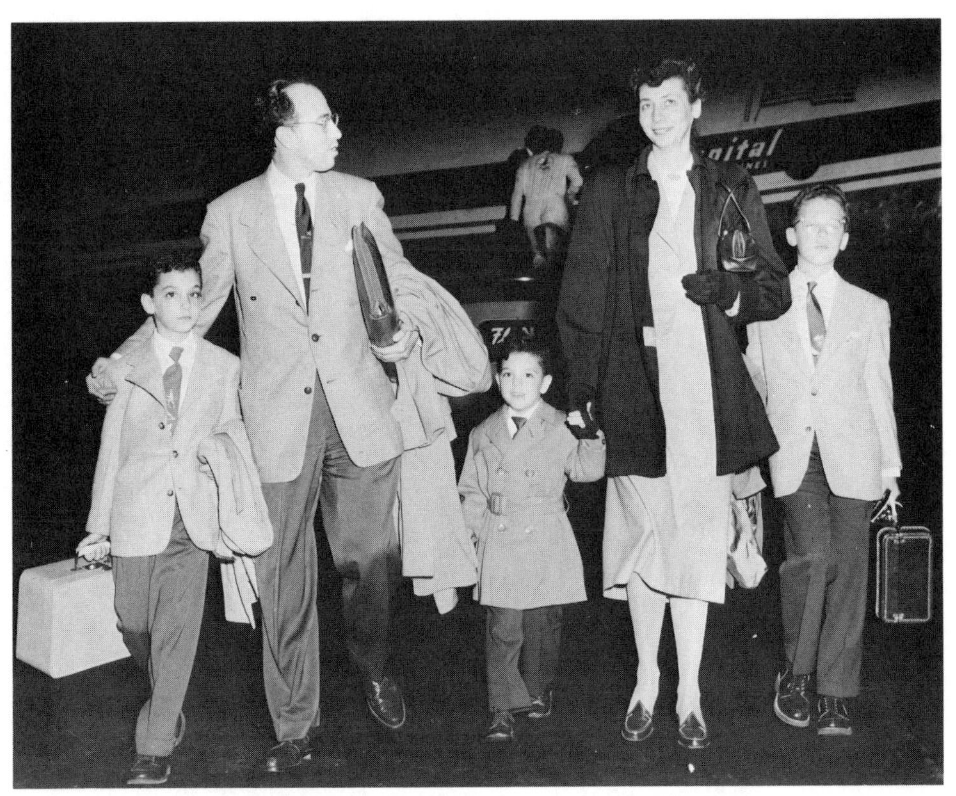

*Arriving in Washington, D.C., to receive a special citation from President Eisenhower, in 1955, Salk is accompanied by his wife, Donna, and their sons: (left to right) Darrell, Jonathan, and Peter.* (AP/Wide World Photos)

# Chapter 5

# A Place for Creative Minds

By 1956, Salk should have been a happy man, but he was not. For every success he had achieved, his detractors had found a way to attack and sidetrack him. Even after the Cutter tragedy had been found to be linked to manufacturing mistakes, even after millions of people had been vaccinated and protected from polio with no ill effects, the scientists and doctors who thought that only a live-virus vaccine would work on polio put roadblocks in the way of Salk's career. Rather than being able to rest on his laurels and move back to his lab, Salk was spending an inordinate amount of his time defending his vaccine and trying to get it distributed to the public.

Salk's one driving motivation during this time was to make sure that his vaccine was used. He did not want people to become paralyzed or even die from a disease for which there was a ready cure. He felt a personal responsibility to make the polio vaccine as widely available as possible.

By 1956, Dr. Albert Sabin and other detractors of Salk's vaccine had stopped criticizing him so aggressively in public, but they did not stop looking for a way to make a live-virus vaccine. They essentially refused to acknowledge Salk's vaccine or dismissed it as a stopgap. Every month, in medical journals, local doctors read that work was continuing on a live-virus vaccine. As a result, many did not make it a priority to get the Salk vaccine to the public. They could not see that a permanent cure for polio was already at hand because it came in a form they had not expected, a killed-virus vaccine. The American Medical Association (AMA), the governing body for doctors in the United States, even went so far as to try and

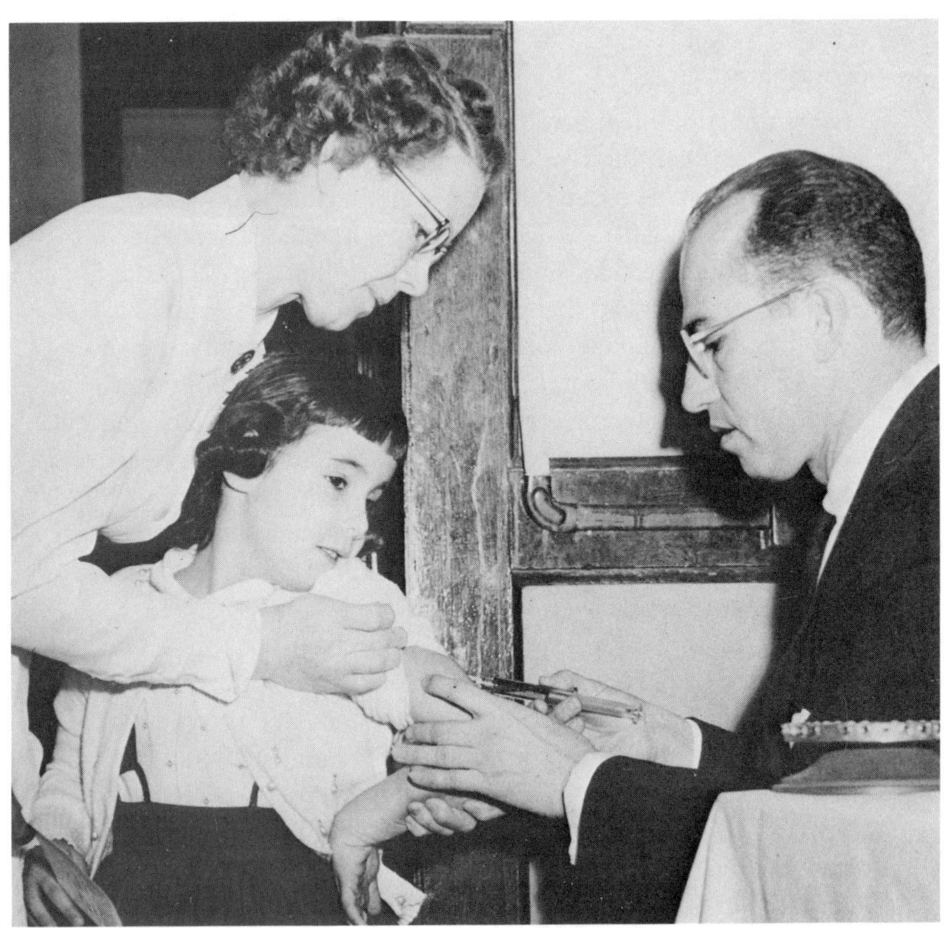

*Salk inoculates six-year-old Deborah Jacobson during a vaccination drive in the Pittsburgh school system in 1956.* (AP/Wide World Photos)

block free distribution of Salk's polio vaccine by the March of Dimes.

When the March of Dimes asked Salk to help convince people to take the vaccine by speaking to groups throughout the United States, he agreed to take on the challenge. People were suffering needlessly. Salk realized that all his successful work in the lab was in jeopardy of being nullified by what was becoming a political battle. He heard of one instance where a doctor was charging five dollars a shot for the polio vaccine—a lot of money in 1956—and turning a tidy profit. "What are you going to do with people like this?" exclaimed Salk. "Six hundred kids who have five dollars get vaccinated, and six hundred who do not have five dollars do not get vaccinated." Salk had worked on his vaccine to conquer polio, not so people could make a profit, and he was stirred to action.

Salk would have preferred to stay in his lab and start work on how cancer affects the immune system, an area he was just becoming interested in, but he agreed to help as he could. He spoke at fund-raisers and luncheons, gave interviews, and wrote articles for journals. His fame and his eloquence assured him an audience.

Because of Salk's help, the campaign to get people vaccinated in 1956 was a success. Celebrities such as Elvis Presley also lent a hand by being inoculated at press events. By the end of the year, thirty million people had been inoculated with Salk's polio vaccine. In 1956, there were 61 percent fewer cases of polio than in 1955. This trend continued for the next couple of years, with most new cases of polio being reported in poorer areas, especially in the poor black neighborhoods of cities where public health services were inadequate.

## Conflicts at Pitt

Events at Salk's home base at the University of Pittsburgh

were also conspiring to make it hard for him to get back to the lab. In the wake of the success of his vaccine, Salk was given the position of head of the new Department of Preventive Medicine at Pitt. He hoped that, as head of his own department, he could sidestep the administrative tangles that had slowed him before. Salk's sudden fame also attracted the attention of a group of wealthy businessmen and women in the local community. These philanthropists pooled funds to buy the wing of the hospital where Salk's basement lab was located and give it to the university. Salk demurred, but the wing was named Salk Hall. There were great expectations that with increased freedom in his research, he would provide the world with more stunning health breakthroughs and the city of Pittsburgh with more fame.

In 1957, however, the university got a new chancellor, Edward Litchfield, who had previously been the president of the Smith-Corona typewriter company. As an administrator, Litchfield sought to exercise strong control over every aspect of the university. While he appreciated Salk's achievements, he refused to give Salk the independence he needed to thrive. Salk realized that after all the hard work he had done to get his freedom at Pitt, he was now back at square one.

Aside from his conflicts with the chancellor, Salk had only limited time to work in his lab in any case. In addition to his duties as a department head at Pitt, he was still forced to spend a great deal of time defending and advocating his vaccine. Despite the overwhelming success of the Salk vaccine, some doctors continued to doubt its effectiveness. Some of Salk's critics even went so far as to suggest that the decrease in polio cases was part of the natural ebb and flow of the disease and that the Salk vaccine had nothing to do with the decrease. In 1961, a letter in the AMA journal said the Salk vaccine was nearly worthless, ignoring the fact that in the five years since the Salk vaccine had been introduced, the number of polio cases per year had decreased by 91 percent.

In 1962, Sabin was ready to introduce his live-virus vaccine. In contrast to Salk, whose killed-virus vaccine challenged long-established medical orthodoxy, Sabin was a representative of the medical mainstream. Moreover, his vaccine did have some advantages over Salk's (see sidebar). The only drawback was that a very small number of people got polio from the Sabin vaccine. Fortunately, such cases were exceedingly rare.

## A New Direction

While the campaign for his vaccine between 1956 and 1960 diverted Salk from the lab, it brought some unexpected benefits as well. At the fund-raising dinners and banquets

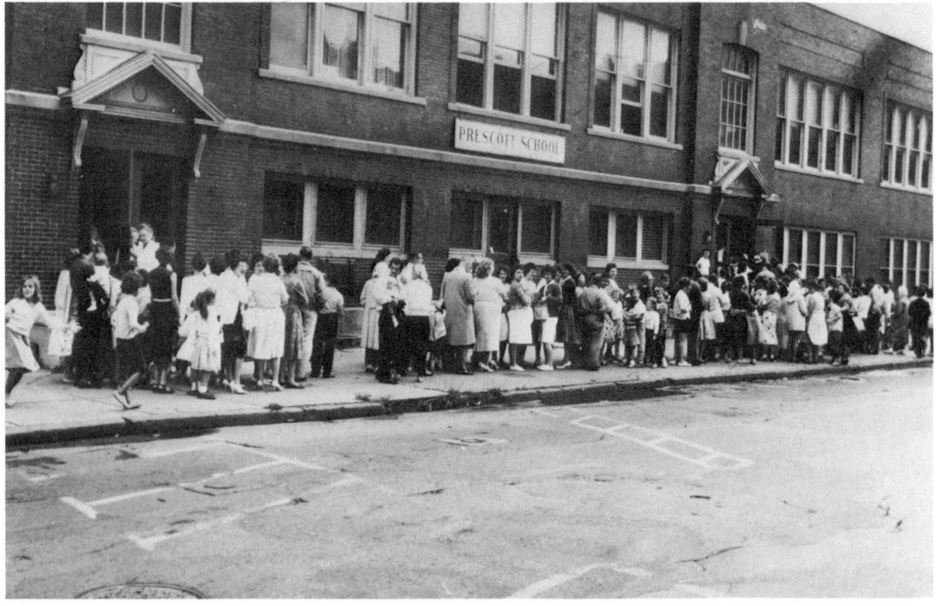


*Crowds line up outside a Syracuse school to receive the Sabin oral polio vaccine in 1961.* AP/Wide World Photos)

which he had to attend for the March of Dimes, Salk was introduced to brilliant people in all sorts of fields. He sat at tables with physicists who had helped to create the atomic bomb, artists who had made great works of art, and psychologists who had plumbed the secrets of the unconscious mind.

**Live-virus vaccine or killed-virus vaccine, Sabin vaccine or Salk vaccine?**

*This is the question faced by doctors and health workers around the world. Both have advantages and disadvantages. The Salk vaccine is safer since it causes no infection, but it is more expensive to produce and administer because it is given in shots. In addition, a certain number of people will always be hesitant to receive an injection, even when it seems clearly in their best interest. In contrast, the relatively inexpensive Sabin vaccine is orally administered, usually in a sugar cube.*

*Approximately one in four million doses of Sabin vaccine causes paralytic polio. However, most people given the Sabin vaccine not only remain healthy but also give peripheral immunity to unvaccinated people who come in contact with them.*

*The Sabin vaccine is overwhelmingly the vaccine of choice in Third World countries. The Salk vaccine continues to be used successfully in developed nations such as Sweden.*

The exposure to all these interesting people and their ideas stimulated Salk's imagination and made the battles that he was engaged in seem small and limited. They opened his mind to a world where he might not have to spend his energy on tasks such as politicking for his vaccine and maintaining his position at Pitt. Salk began to wonder why it was that fields such as physics, biology, and chemistry were separated. They had so much in common. Why couldn't insights from these fields and others be brought together to provide a unified understanding of the human condition?

By 1960, many of Salk's detractors were crowing that he was a one-hit wonder. It had been five years since his vaccine had been released, and what had he done since? Of course, Salk saw things differently. "The incredible experience with the polio vaccine made it possible for me to think in terms of something beyond preventive medicine, beyond a department of microbiology, beyond routine virus research," he said with characteristic optimism. "So a negative situation had led to something positive. Which led to something negative—the promise of an institute of experimental medicine in Pittsburgh collapsed. I thought for a while of simply returning to my work, just as if nothing at all had happened, but the attraction of the biological institute concept was too powerful. An institute of the kind I had been discussing with [nuclear physicists] Leo Szilard and Robert Oppenheimer and other people of minds of scope seemed essential to the rapid progress of biology at this juncture in the history of man."

An institute such as Salk envisioned had never been attempted before. Salk wanted to have scientists working next door to artists and philosophers, free of the constraints and the academic infighting that had hobbled his efforts in Pittsburgh. He wanted to hold meetings with these great minds on all the problems of humankind. In a candid moment, Salk also acknowledged the wear and tear he had experienced since his immersion into public life. "I sometimes think that the idea of creating the institute was to create a shelter for myself."

## The Salk Institute

Just as he had done with his vaccine, Salk turned to Basil O'Connor and the March of Dimes to help him turn his vision into reality. O'Connor liked Salk's idea of an interdisciplinary research center that would be "dedicated to contributing, from the powerful base of modern biology, toward the advancement of the health and well-being of man." He pledged fifteen million dollars to build the initial facility.

During the next couple of years while on their travels to and from March of Dimes events around the country, Salk and O'Connor kept their eyes open for a good spot for the institute. They eventually settled on a site near La Jolla, California, on a bluff overlooking the ocean. As luck would have it, the mayor of nearby San Diego had contracted polio as a child and thus was particularly sympathetic to Salk's vision. In 1960, the city of San Diego donated the land for the institute, and Salk announced that he was leaving Pitt to become the founding director of an as yet unnamed and unbuilt research center.

Salk wanted the facilities of his institute to represent its founding ideals; he wanted the buildings to be practical laboratories, but also beautiful and inspiring. He enlisted the help of Philadelphia architect Louis Kahn to design the institute. The working relationship between Salk and Kahn soon blossomed into another of the long line of creative pairings that Salk has made over his lifetime. Salk became Kahn's "most trusted critic and favorite client." The two men shared the view that all disciplines are complementary and bring out the best in each other. This proved true of their relationship as well. The result of their collaboration is considered a masterpiece of modern architecture.

When construction was completed in 1963, the center was christened the Salk Institute for Biological Studies. It was named thus at O'Connor's insistence; in his modesty, Salk would have omitted his own name. The main building of this "temple of science" consists of two almost identical wings that house lab quarters, called the "served space" by Kahn. The lab quarters can be used for many different kinds of research. They can accommodate the huge vats of frozen nitrogen used in freezing immune-system cells so that DNA can be separated from them, leading to a greater understanding of how the body protects itself against infection. The labs have also housed computer banks used in pioneering studies that analyze how humans move.

All pipes, wires, bulky lab machines, and other mechanical and maintenance materials are located between the lab floors in the area that Kahn designated as "servant space." This allows the lab space itself to remain unencumbered. The two enormous wings are separated by a cement courtyard that looks over the cliffs to the ocean, to the western horizon and its stunning sunsets. A narrow canal runs down the center of the courtyard. Salk says it represents the life force in all things. At certain times of the day the whole institute glows with a pinkish aura, as if it were alive. The glow doesn't come from the work that takes place inside, as it might seem, but from the cement Kahn used for the building: a kind the Romans invented that absorbs sunlight.

Now that Salk had an institute, he had to find scientists to fill it. Besides working with Kahn on designing the building, Salk had spent the three years since he left Pitt recruiting some of the world's most respected scientists to come and work at the institute. He lured them with offers that seemed almost too good to be true. All the resident scientists would be given lab space and money to spend on any type of research they chose. They would have complete control over their experiments. If they were doing research on brain tumors and suddenly decided it would be better to work on athlete's foot, they could change direction at will. They were not required to do any teaching or administrative work and did not have to answer to anyone.

The first Fellows of the institute included several Nobel laureates. Dr. Francis Crick and Dr. Renato Dulbecco received Nobel prizes for helping discover the molecular structure of

DNA. Dr. Salvador Luria and Dr. Jacques Monod explained how cells make proteins out of raw materials. All the scientists had diverse interests. Dr. Jacob Bronowski was a mathematician who used his math skills in anthropological studies and was also an authority on the poet William Blake. Salk personally sought out, met with, and convinced each Fellow to come to the institute.

The Salk Institute opened in 1963 with a great deal of media hoopla. Headlines proclaimed that Salk had created a place where countless breakthroughs would be made. *Life* magazine ran two articles on Salk and the institute, newspapers ran front-page stories, and television gave lots of air time to Salk's new triumph.

However, as with his vaccine, the honeymoon was short-lived. While people liked the idea of the institute, Salk found that it was difficult to sustain funding for his visionary goals. The meetings of artists, scientists, and political leaders on issues crucial to the human condition—issues such as world hunger and overcrowding—had to be shelved. The cross-pollination that Salk had envisioned never really took off. Dr. Bronowski's widely acclaimed television series, "The Ascent of Man," which detailed the evolution of science through human history, was the only major interdisciplinary project to come from the institute in its first years, and it was coproduced by the British Broadcasting Corporation.

When Salk was able to obtain major funding, much of it came with the stipulation that it be used exclusively for cancer research. This important research continues to the present day, but the restrictions meant that the institute was not offering the extraordinary creative freedom that Salk had hoped to provide. Moreover, Salk again found himself spending enormous chunks of his time on fund-raising instead of research.

## A Fresh Start

Salk's life was changing in other ways, too. In 1968, he and his wife Donna were divorced after twenty-eight years of marriage. Fame and the public life the Salks were forced into because of Jonas' position at the institute put strains on family life. The years of public scrutiny and time apart eventually proved too much. Donna was becoming increasingly involved in social work again, now that the children were nearly grown, and she resented the obstacles her husband's fame put in her own life. She had been able to put up with Jonas' eighteen-hour-days while he was working on the polio

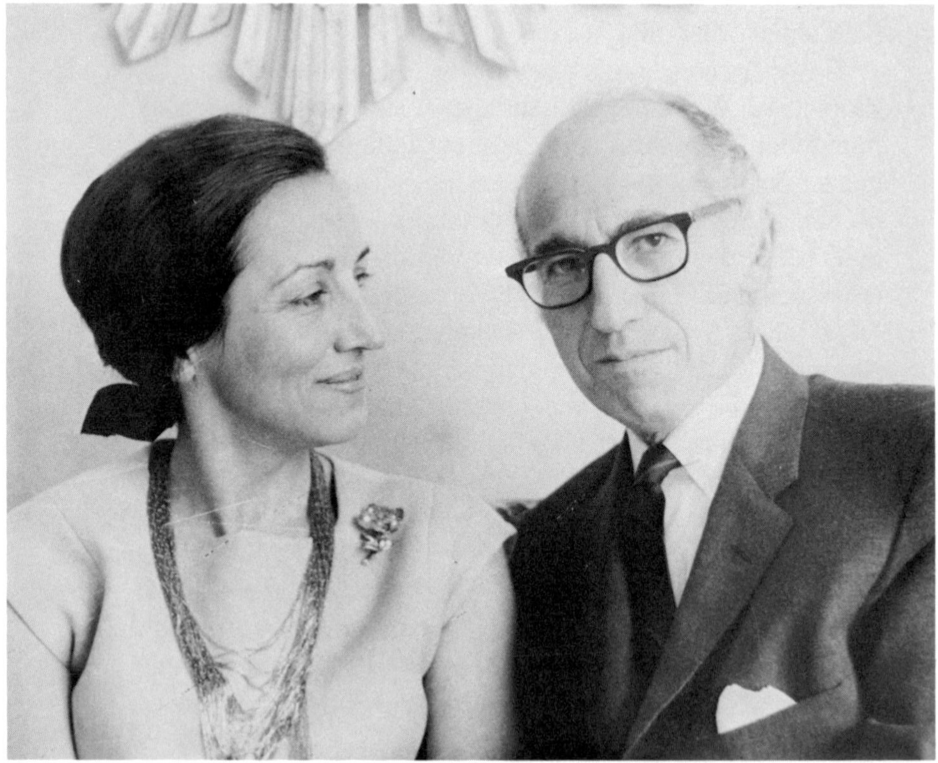

*Salk and Françoise Gilot, shortly before their marriage in 1970.* (AP/Wide World Photos)

vaccine, but now she saw him just as little and there was no tangible goal in sight—nothing but an endless round of fund-raising and administrative work. Like many other couples, Jonas and Donna Salk found themselves going in different directions.

In 1969, Salk was fifty-five years old and ready for another challenge. In his few spare moments, ideas were coming to him that did not quite fit into his role as research scientist and administrator. The institute was generally being hailed as a success, even though it had not lived up to Salk's perfectionist hopes, but Salk was becoming edgy again. He was not ready to assume the role of an elder statesman. He felt like he was stagnating.

The spark Salk needed came in 1970 when he married Françoise Gilot, a talented painter whom he met at a dinner party; one of their first dates was a tour of the institute. Gilot had begun exhibiting her paintings in the finest galleries of France when she was only in her early twenties. In 1943, at the age of eighteen, she had met Pablo Picasso. Although they never married, Gilot and Picasso had two children, Claude (born in 1947) and Paloma (born in 1949).

Picasso was widely regarded as the greatest artist of his time. In his dealings with women he was dominating and often abusive. Unlike his other mistresses and wives, Gilot maintained her independence from Picasso—in part, perhaps, because she was an artist in her own right. In 1964, she wrote a memoir about Picasso that he unsuccessfully tried to suppress. She has also written several other memoirs and studies of artists she has known, including Henri Matisse.

With Gilot, Salk found a mate who matched his creativity and energy, as well as someone who understood the media pressure of fame. Because reporters hounded them, the couple went so far as to sit at different tables in a restaurant in New York before their marriage. To elude the press, they were married in Paris before the announced day.

Shortly after their marriage, Salk stepped down as director of the institute and began working on yet another new project. His ever-questioning mind, now at ease and freed of the responsibilities of administering the institute, turned to larger issues. In 1972, his first book, *Man Unfolding*, was published. Always probing, he was increasingly preoccupied with fundamental questions concerning evolution and the nature of humankind.

# Chapter 6

# AIDS: A New Crusade

In 1984, Salk closed his personal lab at the Salk Institute for Biological Studies. He was seventy years old at the time and it seemed a natural thing to do. He lived in a beautiful home in La Jolla that looked out over the expanse of the Pacific Ocean. His sons were grown and pursuing their own careers: His son Peter had become a research biologist, carrying on the family tradition of medical and scientific excellence; his son Jonathan had coauthored a book of philosophy with him. Salk had spent five decades working on various scientific problems, written four books on philosophy and hundreds of scientific papers, founded the Salk Institute, and discovered the first successful vaccine for polio. Why not make room for another scientist at the institute? Why not retire and take life at a slower pace?

For Salk, however, sitting still was easier said than done. By the mid-1980's, researchers throughout the world were struggling to understand the AIDS virus. Salk simply could not remain on the sidelines while others were searching for the tools to fight this deadly global epidemic. In April, 1987, Salk and his associates began experiments with four chimpanzees to test theories he had developed about ways to combat the AIDS virus. Several months later he published his AIDS theories and the details of his experiment in a British journal, *Nature.*

## An Evolutionary Perspective

Beyond the great compassion that always motivated his actions, Salk had spent the previous fifteen years developing a personal philosophy that almost required him to work on AIDS. Salk had been having trouble sleeping for many years,

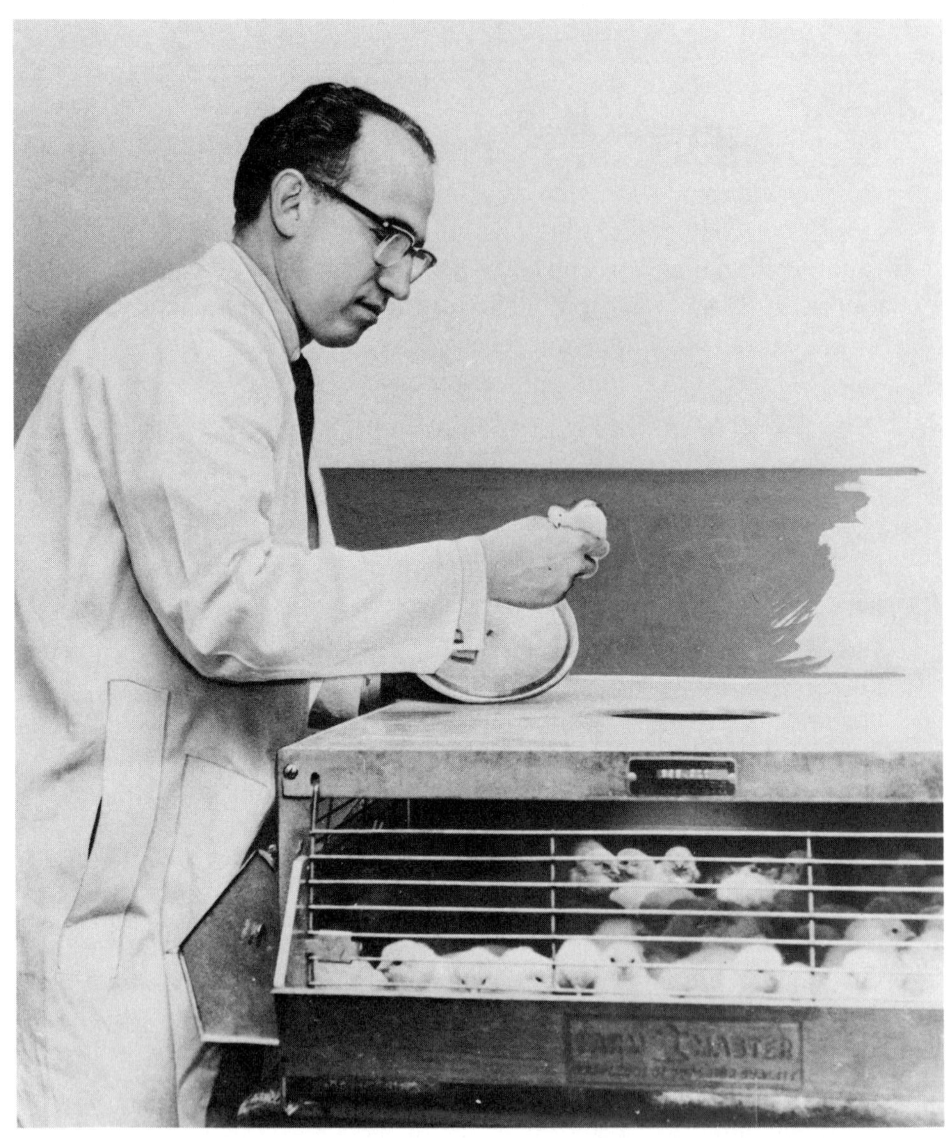

*Salk examines some of the chicks used in experiments at his lab in 1959.* (AP/Wide World Photos)

not because he worried or suffered from insomnia, but because it seemed that whenever he closed his eyes, ideas came to him. A sense of urgency would overcome Salk at such moments—a sense that something larger than himself, the force of evolution, was behind these ideas, that they might hold some clue for making the human condition better. He felt that he had to get up and write these ideas down or lose them forever.

Often in the darkest part of the night, Salk will rise and go to his study and work on what he calls his "night writing." Writing in longhand, Salk fills notebooks with wide-ranging speculations: why the human population is growing so rapidly, how the mind works, how life and ideas evolve, and what the best course for the future of humankind will be. Ideas from these writing sessions became the basis for the four books of philosophy he has published.

Salk's philosophical ideas come from his own life experiences, but they are based on the theories of Charles Darwin, the nineteenth-century biologist who explained the process of evolution. Darwin said that animals which have the best traits for survival in an environment—the ability to run fast, for example, or skin that camouflages them—will survive and reproduce, thus passing their traits on to their offspring via their genes. Conversely, animals which do not have advantageous traits will be more likely to die before they reproduce.

Salk took Darwin's idea and broadened it to apply to more than just animal life. "In its broadest meaning, the concept of universal evolution attempts to unify all that exists," he states in his book *Anatomy of Reality.* Salk hypothesizes that there is a force of evolution, expressed in what we call scientific laws, that caused the dust from space to form into the more complex matter of stars and planets and eventually into living things. He proposes that this force of evolution is in everything and expresses itself in the intricate patterns of the natural world.

Salk also theorizes that at each stage of evolution, there is a critical dilemma or conflict between two complementary forms, a binary relationship, and that this is the primary form evolution takes. For instance, he says that one binary relationship in evolution is the tension between the desires and necessities of an individual and what the species or society requires of that individual. Another example is the binary relationship between the mind and the body.

Salk believes that, with the emergence of human beings, evolution has reached a new stage. For the first time, the vehicles of evolution are capable of understanding their place in the evolutionary march. While he believes that it is a genetically selected trait for human beings to care for one another and take an active role in furthering their evolution, he feels that some people are more aware of their place in evolution than others. Those who are more in tune with evolution, Salk believes, should be nurtured so they can develop into the great scientists, artists, and leaders of humankind. Furthermore, he believes that it is the responsibility of these exceptional individuals, selected randomly by evolution, to lead humankind to a higher level of evolution, avoiding the routes that would lead to extinction.

These ideas, in a less developed form, led to the founding of the Salk Institute for Biological Studies. In the 1970's and 1980's, when nuclear war seemed to be a very real possibility, Salk worked out his philosophy of hope and evolution to help show the way toward a peaceful and profitable existence.

These convictions gave Salk a special sense of responsibility when the AIDS virus appeared, and a unique perspective on the disease. "I assume there has to be a solution to the AIDS problem," Salk said. "I say that because of the recognition that this is an evolutionary struggle between two evolving forces. The AIDS virus has evolved mechanisms to defy the systems that exist within us to eliminate it. It has

*There is a new reality—that man is a part of the cosmos and that, just as the individual cell needs the organism of which he is a part, mankind needs—and therefore cannot destroy—his world. I think that awareness of man's place in the universe is growing. But I also believe that those in policy-making positions need to develop a greater appreciation of the reality we are talking about. We must understand that it is not just that the world looks different; it is different. The world is different because it is infinitely more crowded than it was back when human evolution first began. We are different because our knowledge and power have increased to the point that we have it within our power to destroy the very planet on which we live. We're going to have to rely on artists as well as scientists for the solutions we need, people who want to visualize the architecture of human relationships.* [Jonas Salk, "A Conversation with Jonas Salk," *Psychology Today* 16 (March, 1983)]

outsmarted us thus far. But I cannot believe that we are not smart enough to find a way at least to work out a negotiated peace or a settlement involving live and let live."

## "AIDS Is Different": Doubters Again

Salk moved on AIDS with the speed and efficiency that he had shown in his path-breaking polio work, reorganizing existing ideas to apply to a new problem and searching for a fast solution to save lives. In 1987, Salk began taking whole HIV viruses and killing them with formalin to make a vaccine, much as he had for polio.

The majority of Salk's scientific peers viewed his approach to AIDS with skepticism. All the potential problems of a killed-virus vaccine were dredged up again, in addition to other objections. As he had done with polio, Salk attacked

AIDS in a way that challenged the assumptions of the scientific mainstream.

Unlike normal vaccines that try to prevent disease before it happens, Salk's work on AIDS is targeted for people who already have tested positive for the HIV virus. He calls the idea immunotherapy. Diseases such as rabies and hepatitis are controlled with a similar technique called passive immunity. Unlike most viruses, which cause disease quickly after entering the body, the HIV virus attaches itself to a cell and then lies dormant for several years before it causes AIDS. Salk figures that if you can help the body recognize cells harboring the HIV virus, the immune system can kill these cells and perhaps hold off AIDS indefinitely.

"The idea is to prevent disease now, even in the presence of infection—to see if we can intervene early, before the symptoms arise," said Salk in an interview in 1990. "I'm only interested in solving the problem, and I don't care how. My style is old-fashioned. I don't know how else to do it. I have nothing to contribute from a molecular biological point of view [genetic engineering]—it's not my field. My job is to inactivate the virus and present it in a form that will trick the immune system into reacting."

Most other AIDS researchers doubt that Salk's techniques will work. They point out that the HIV virus is much more complex than the polio virus. There are at least twenty known types of the HIV virus, and, to make things more complex, HIV mutates often and dramatically. Many researchers believe that the most effective way to combat HIV will be to use genetic engineering techniques to isolate the bits and pieces of the HIV virus that the immune system reacts against. These noninfectious pieces of the virus could then be used to trick the immune system into developing antibodies in the blood for the HIV virus. The majority of scientists working on AIDS see Salk's work as complementary to their work because it tells

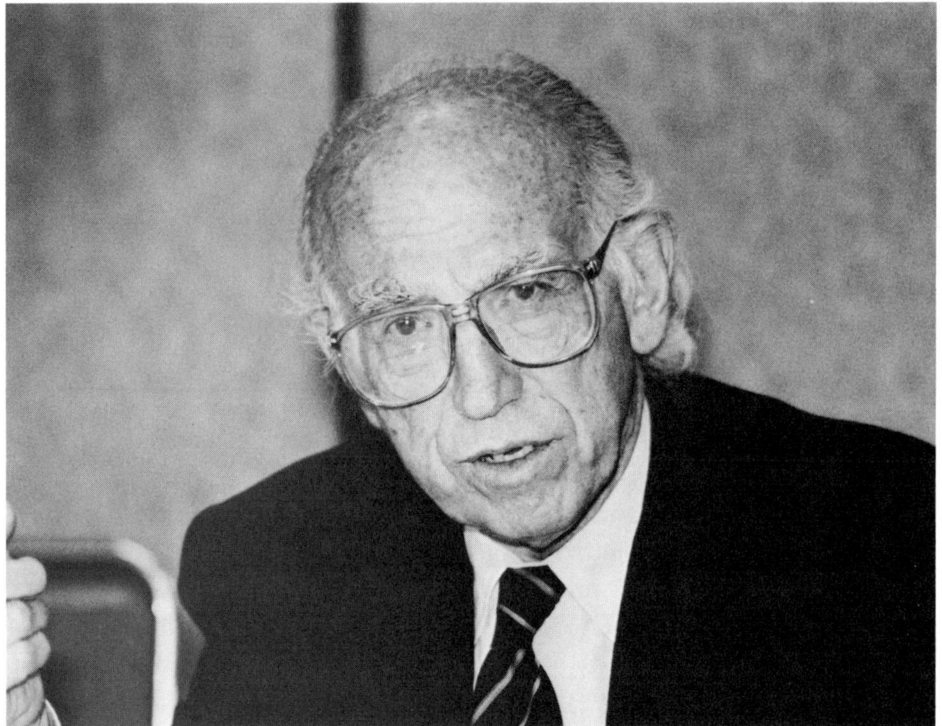

*Salk in 1991 speaks with reporters in Seattle about his AIDS research.* (AP/Wide World Photos)

them more about how the HIV virus functions. However, they do not think Salk's hypothesis of passive resistance is the way that AIDS will be controlled.

## Positive Results

Despite the naysayers, Salk's early tests with monkeys were successful. In 1987, Salk's collaborator, Dr. Clarence Gibbs, injected two chimpanzees with killed HIV to stimulate their immune systems and then later injected the chimps with live HIV to test their immunity. The chimps remained virus-free, suggesting that they had developed antibodies for HIV.

As soon as his monkey test showed results in 1987, Salk

began to push for human tests of his preparation. Only in humans can one really assess how a vaccine meant for humans will work. However, jumping from tests on monkeys to tests on humans was not as easy in 1987 as it had been in 1951, when Salk simply went to a school or prison and got permission from the principal or warden to use their wards as test subjects. After the Cutter incident in 1955, state and federal governments had taken a much more active role in monitoring scientific tests, especially tests of potentially harmful drugs and vaccines.

Nevertheless, Salk managed to move through the inspections and piles of paperwork with unusual speed, and he was given permission by California state health officials and the federal Food and Drug Administration to test the safety of his HIV preparation on people already infected with HIV. This way, if the preparation was not safe, it would not cause someone who was HIV-negative to become infected. In November of 1987, Salk's collaborator, Dr. Alexandra Levine in Los Angeles, gave eighty-two volunteers who were HIV-positive the killed-virus preparation to test its safety. If the preparation was safe, it wouldn't increase the advent of AIDS. Two years later, the volunteers were as healthy as they had been when they received the preparation, and many of the volunteers' antibody levels had gone up, suggesting that besides being safe, the preparation helped prevent the onset of AIDS.

By 1990, Salk was hoping to test the effectiveness of his preparation by giving it to healthy people. He wanted to stimulate their antibody reaction and then extract these antibodies and inject them into people who were HIV-positive. The healthy people would function as an antibody factory, Salk hypothesized. In an effort to find willing test subjects, Salk contacted the Catholic Church in the Archdiocese of Los Angeles and asked if priests or nuns would be interested in helping in the project.

The media somehow found out about Salk's inquiry, and he was instantly enveloped in a media circus similar to what he had experienced with his polio vaccine. Headlines screamed that Salk would be testing a full-blown AIDS vaccine on priests and nuns. Recognizing Salk's name and recalling his past success, the public began to raise its hopes. However, Salk was much more savvy in his old age and was able to convince the press that he was not far enough along in his project to warrant the attention he was getting.

## Still Questioning

Behind the media blitz, Salk was finding results to his tests that he had not expected. Only about half of the HIV-positive volunteers who had been injected with his killed-virus preparation were developing antibodies in their bloodstream. Normally, this would be considered a failure in a test of a vaccine. However, Salk noticed that the other patients, the ones who were not developing antibodies, were actually resisting the onset of AIDS more effectively than the test subjects who had developed antibodies. Poring over his notes from the experiment, he noticed that when the people who had not developed antibodies had been injected with the killed HIV virus, they had developed a small rash or reddening of the skin where the needle had gone into them. At first, Salk could not explain what this meant, but he tucked the information in his memory and kept his eyes open.

One day, while he was reading an article in a scientific journal about some studies of leprosy, an answer came to Salk. Researchers had found that resistance to leprosy was associated with an early immune-system response to an infection called the TH1 stage. In the TH1 stage, the immune system produces cells called T-cells that cannibalize infected cells. Normally, the immune system moves past the TH1 stage relatively quickly to the TH2 stage, when it begins making antibodies for the blood. In the leprosy study, patients with antibodies in their bloodstream gave into the disease more quickly than those without antibodies.

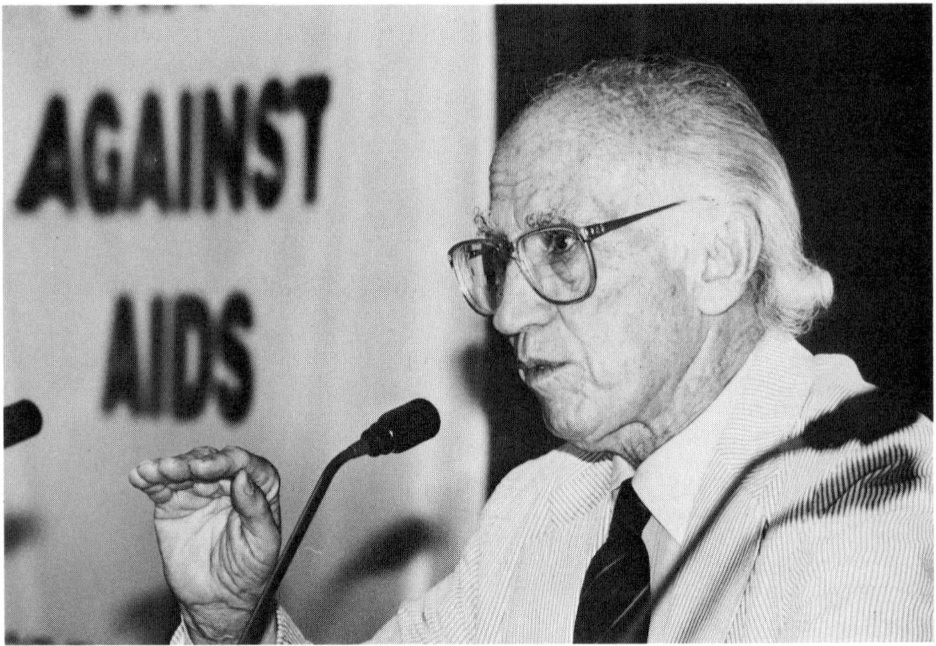


*Salk holds a press conference at the Eighth Annual International Conference on AIDS, held in Amsterdam in 1992.* (AP/Wide World Photos)

Salk realized that his experiments had produced the same results, although obviously with a different disease. His study of evolution had drawn his attention to the fact that all living creatures share structures. If leprosy and the HIV virus cause the same reaction in the body, Salk hypothesized, it is likely that leprosy and HIV are structured similarly. In support of his hunch, Salk noted that one of the characteristics of the TH1 response is a rash or wheal on the skin. Now that he knew where to look, Salk was able to find several other studies that had similar results. "The curtain just went down," he said of his inspiration.

In July of 1992, Salk went to the eighth annual AIDS conference in Amsterdam and presented his new theory. He announced that almost all current AIDS research is misguided because it works toward developing an antibody response from the body. Salk's theory holds that the way to prevent AIDS will be to keep the body from producing antibodies because the production of antibodies stops the production of T-cells, which seem to be most effective in preventing the advancement of AIDS. He acknowledged that he did not yet know how to stall the immune system in the TH1 stage, but that was the direction he was now pursuing. He said he thought exposure to a very tiny amount of the HIV virus might be the best way to cause a freeze in the TH1 stage.

Salk's audacity angered many of the other scientists at the conference. He was calling into question the work of the leading researchers in the field. Salk's critics accused him of creating "the maximum amount of speculation from a minimum amount of data." Nevertheless, when the conference ended, Salk's ideas were being seriously debated, even if they were not popular. The years ahead will show whether Salk's latest work is as successful as his earlier projects.

# Chapter 7

# Salk's Legacy

Jonas Salk's life and work have meant many different things to many different people. He is proof of the subjectivity of history. To some he is a hero and to others he is a blasphemer. In either case, it is hard to put a lid on Salk's career. In his old age he continues to do important work, and many of his past projects are still bearing fruit. He will, inevitably, be best remembered as the man who found a cure for polio. However, in his personal time line polio was really only a stepping-off point.

Salk's work and life fused into one entity after he discovered his polio vaccine, and he became focused on larger issues concerning the health and vitality of humankind. His work at any given time was always built upon what he had done previously. Ironically, this eventually led him full circle, from his polio vaccine work, through his work on more abstract projects such as the Salk Institute and his books, and then back to lab work on another deadly affliction, AIDS.

Salk is definitely a hero to his family. For years after the fact, Jonas' father, Daniel, carried in his wallet copies of news clips from April 12, 1955, announcing the success of the Salk vaccine. Daniel was so proud of his son that wherever he went he showed the clips to anyone who was interested. Daniel saw his own success in his children's achievements. All three of his sons attained success in their careers, but Jonas' fame as a saver of lives and conqueror of disease was a special fulfillment of the dreams that had motivated Daniel Salk's sacrifices on behalf of his family.

In turn, Jonas Salk's own children came to respect and

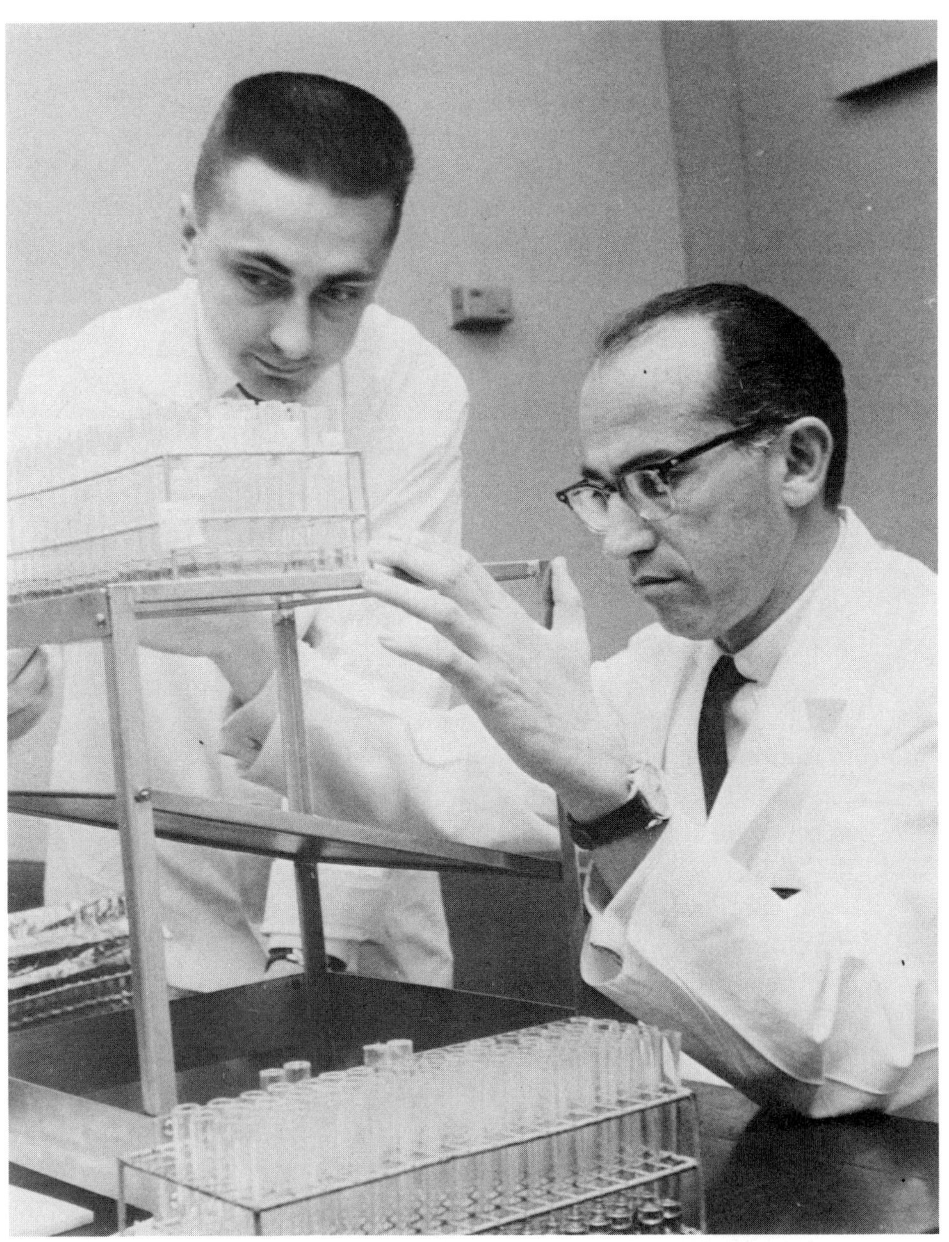

*Salk in 1959 in his lab at the University of Pittsburgh, with his colleague Abel Prinzie of Belgium.* (AP/Wide World Photos)

honor him; they, too, chose to enter the medical profession. His son Peter was skeptical of his father's ideas on AIDS but also showed that he understood and respected his father. "I thought it [his father's approach to AIDS] was crazy. . . . But he just had this idea that he kept before him and it has allowed him to gather all the things that he developed over the years and put them together in a way that absolutely no one else, to my awareness, is capable of doing," Peter told a reporter for *Life* magazine in 1990. All the members of the Salk family have respected Jonas' desire to keep his personal life, and the rest of the family members' lives, private and out of the media.

## Contrasting Views

Among the general public, Salk will be recognized as a member of the popular pantheon of doctors and scientists who have saved millions of lives and improved the human race's standard of living through work in the microscopic realm of disease prevention. In September of 1992, the Pan American Health Organization announced that there had not been a case of polio reported in the Western Hemisphere for more than a year. Polio has been eliminated from the Americas, and there is hope that it will be eliminated worldwide before the year 2000. Salk is responsible for this, even if many of the people were vaccinated with the Sabin vaccine. Salk's bravado in developing his vaccine, and his understanding of its importance in human terms, pushed up the time when an effective polio vaccine would be available by at least ten years. Salk acted as a catalyst for other scientists in making his vaccine.

The scientists Salk pushed did not like being pushed. Many of them had built their careers by moving methodically over complex scientific problems in a tightly sealed world consisting only of test tubes and other scientists. Salk's unfaltering confidence in himself and his work was another

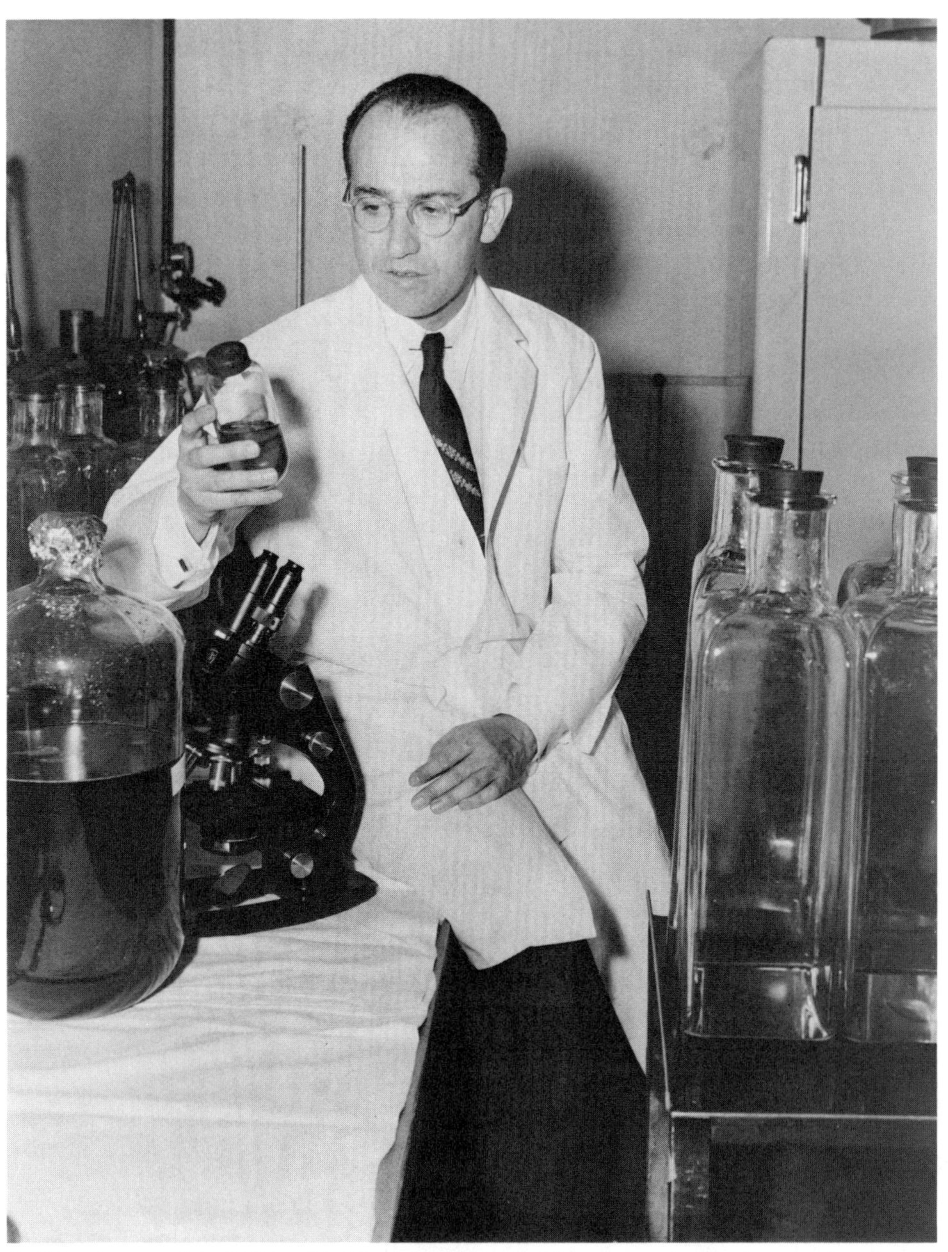

*Salk back at work in 1955 at his Municipal Hospital laboratory in Pittsburgh after the announcement of his successful polio vaccine.* (AP/Wide World Photos)

reason he offended many scientists. Furthermore, many scientists saw Salk's polio work as only a refinement of previously invented techniques and thus unworthy of attention and certainly not worthy of the media hype it received. In 1990, thirty-five years after the Salk vaccine became a reality, Dr. Sabin was still attacking Salk. "It was pure kitchen chemistry," he told a *New York Times* writer. "Salk didn't discover anything."

For these reasons Salk will be remembered in two different ways for a single event. While the average citizen sees Salk as a saver of lives, many in the scientific community despise Salk because they see him as a threat to their way of working and to the scientific ideals of research medicine. Many scientists use Salk as an example of someone who did not know his place and did not avoid the limelight, as befits a scientist. However, Salk was the first of his kind of researcher and had to be brash to accomplish what he did. The tragedy for Salk is that he lost the respect of many of his peers by advancing science into the consciousness of society at large.

## Monument to a Visionary

In fifty years the politics and egos of the polio vaccine debate will be footnotes in history books, but the Salk Institute of Biological Studies will remain etched against the horizon on the cliffs of La Jolla. Many famous people have monuments built to honor their achievements. The majority of these statues gather rust and pigeons as they slowly decay and are forgotten. It is fitting that the closest thing to a monument to Salk is a living, creative research institute.

The institute is the most tangible expression of Salk's ideas and his life's work. The institute is a place where all things are possible and all facets of existence are deemed important. Written into the institute's charter, and designed into the buildings, is an understanding that questioning why something is done is as important as actually doing it.

After the institute, Salk turned to trying to assimilate all his life experiences and all the knowledge he had accumulated into a framework where it all made sense. Salk's philosophical books are proving to be more and more pertinent as the years pass. They are finding their expression in the more progressive projects and policies of institutions around the world. His emphasis on interdisciplinary studies is finding an echo in the way many colleges design their courses and the way businesses work. His theories concerning population growth may or may not prove true, but they are a useful tool in talking about the problem. His perspective on evolution and the progression of knowledge is equally provocative. His recognition of the global threats posed by unwise human activities, from pollution to the nuclear arms-race, contributed to our growing awareness of environmental issues.

It is a strange twist of fate that Salk's philosophical ideas helped turn him toward AIDS research. At a basic emotional level, his theorizing that some people have special skills that can help humankind and that these people are obligated to help may simply be a rationalization of his compassion for human suffering. Some might suggest that it is a little egotistical for Salk to decide that he is in a position to have an important bearing on the problems of humankind, but in the case of AIDS it turns out he actually is in that position. It is too early to say whether or not Salk's work on AIDS will provide an answer to the problem. History will certainly note that he was a contributor to the solution of yet another major dilemma of humankind during his lifetime.

Above and beyond all debate on the merits of Salk's various projects, this proves true: Salk was always able to identify the major problems of his time and throw his weight into solving these problems. If his theories about AIDS and population growth prove correct and if the Salk Institute continues to

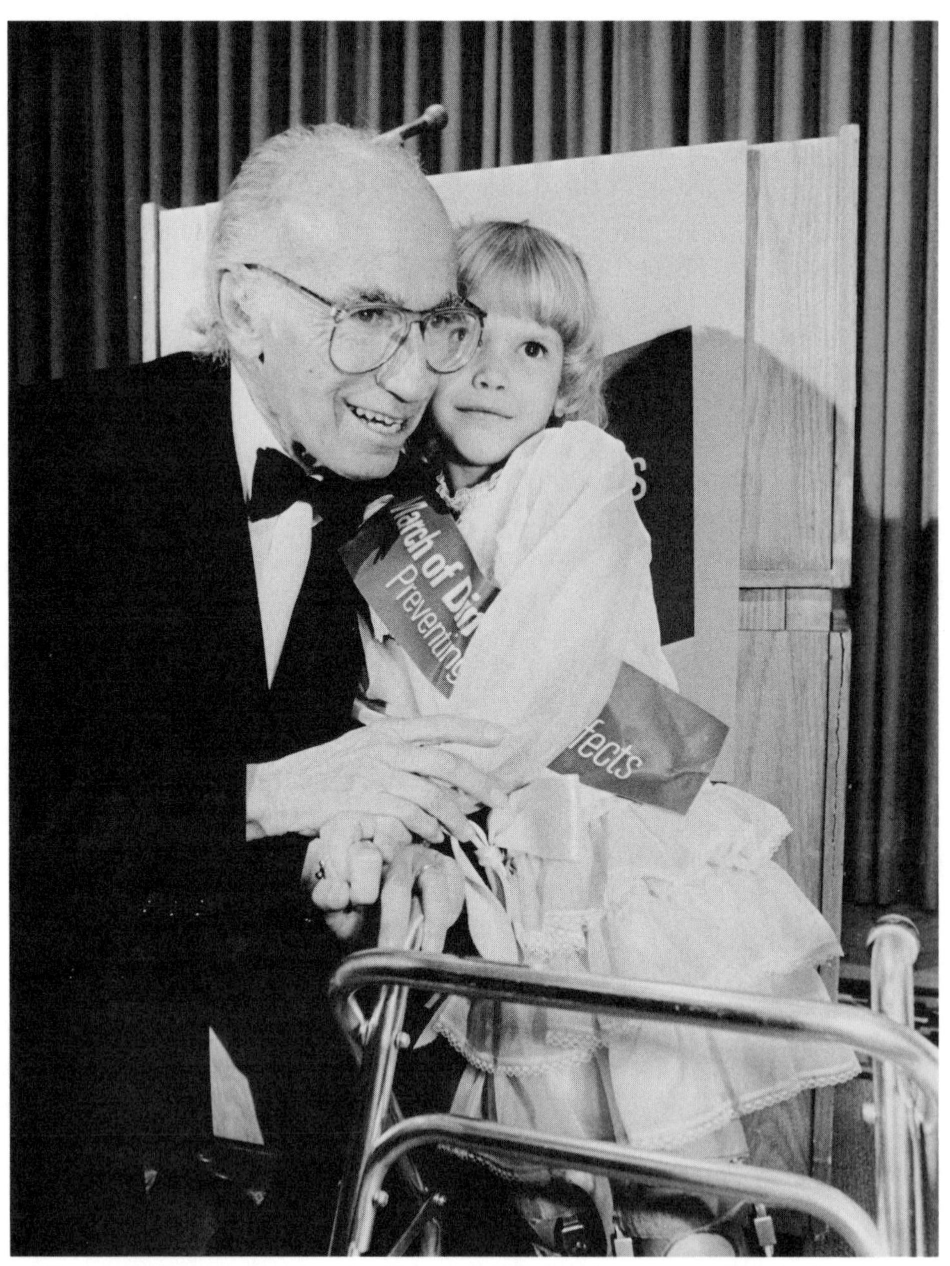

*Salk's legacy; the occasion was the 30th anniversary of the creation of the Salk vaccine.*
(AP/Wide World Photos)

prosper and produce quality scientific research, Salk may well be hailed as a renaissance man of the twentieth century. Whether or not his theories are validated, however, Salk's work ethic and his compassion for the plight of the human race mark him as someone who is worthy of emulation.

# Viruses

Polio is only one of the countless viruses discovered by modern science. These submicroscopic parasites affect our lives in many ways, from the recurring nuisance of the common cold to the immeasurable impact of the worldwide AIDS epidemic.

While AIDS is the viral disease that currently poses the greatest challenge to researchers, virologists are waging a never-ending war on many fronts. The influenza or flu virus, for example, is troubling because of its ability to mutate rapidly. This year's flu vaccine won't be effective against next year's virus. Normally, however miserable its effects may be, the flu virus is not fatal, but occasionally a particularly virulent strain evolves. More than twenty million people died in the worldwide flu epidemic of 1918.

The study of viruses began in response to specific diseases, and the prevention of disease is still virology's primary mission. At the same time, however, by studying viruses researchers are learning more about the basic building blocks within the living cell.

Listed below are several sources that provide a good introduction to viruses and virology. For sources that focus on the polio virus, the polio vaccines, and Jonas Salk's life and work as a whole, see the Bibliography that follows.

Guidici, Ann Fettner. *Viruses: Agents of Change*. New York: McGraw-Hill, 1990. A straightforward overview, intended for the general reader.

Henig, Robin Marantz. *A Dancing Matrix: Voyages Along the Viral Frontier*. New York: Alfred A. Knopf, 1993. This provocative book conveys both the daunting challenge of viral disease and the excitement of virologists' pathbreaking research in genetic engineering, by means of which they hope to trick viruses into bolstering the body's immune system. Warning against complacency, Henig suggests that another worldwide flu epidemic is likely to strike before the end of the twentieth century.

Levine, Arnold J. *Viruses*. New York: Scientific American Library,

1992. A superbly illustrated state-of-the-art introduction, accessible to the general reader.

Preston, Richard. "Crisis in the Hot Zone." *The New Yorker* 68 (October 26, 1992): 58-81. A compulsively readable narrative that recalls Michael Crichton's classic thriller *The Andromeda Strain*, this article focuses on "hot agents": deadly viruses for which, in most cases, no vaccine or cure has yet been developed. Incursion into the tropics is bringing humans into widespread contact with viruses that have been evolving in relative isolation for aeons; many of these viruses are lethal. Along the way Preston provides an introduction to viruses that is worth textbook treatments ten times as long.

# Time Line

| | |
|---|---|
| 1914 | Jonas Salk is born in New York City. |
| 1939 | Graduation from NYU Medical School. Begins his association with Dr. Thomas Francis and his work toward an influenza vaccine. |
| 1940 | Jonas Salk and Donna Lindsay are married. Salk begins his internship at Mt. Sinai Hospital in New York. |
| 1942 | Moves to the University of Michigan to work full-time on an influenza vaccine with Dr. Francis. Until 1945, works closely with the U.S. Army to prevent influenza epidemics on military bases across the world. |
| 1947 | Leaves Michigan to become director of the newly created University of Pittsburgh Virus Research Lab. |
| 1949 | Begins poliomyelitis typing studies for the March of Dimes. Dr. John Enders develops a way to cultivate polio virus in test tubes; Salk is the first to utilize in practical applications. |
| 1952 | Tests killed-virus vaccine first on himself, then on his family and in limited field studies at the Polk State School and Watson Home for Crippled Children in Pennsylvania. Against the advice of leading virologists, such as Dr. Albert Sabin, the March of Dimes decides to fund full-scale development of the Salk vaccine. |
| 1954 | Large national field tests of the Salk killed-virus vaccine are conducted by Dr. Thomas Francis working for the March of Dimes to determine the safety and effectiveness of the Salk vaccine. |
| 1955 | The Salk vaccine is approved for public use, and mass production begins. Two weeks after the Salk vaccine is licensed, a batch of vaccine from Cutter Laboratories in Berkeley, California, is found to cause paralytic polio. National hysteria is quelled when the bad vaccine is found to be the result of manufacturing mistakes. |

| | |
|---|---|
| 1956-1961 | Salk enters a time of readjustment to his sudden fame and works to have his vaccine accepted by the public and scientific community. The seeds for the Salk Institute are sown. |
| 1962 | The Salk vaccine is supplanted in general use by the Sabin vaccine, which uses attenuated live viruses. Heated political battles between the supporters of the Salk and Sabin vaccines precede the switch. |
| 1963 | Salk leaves the University of Pittsburgh to become the founding director of the Salk Institute for Biological Studies in La Jolla, California. Lack of funding for the next three decades prevents the institute from realizing all the interdisciplinary and ethical debate programs Salk initially envisioned. |
| 1963-1984 | Salk works on problems of the immune system and cancer in his lab at the institute. |
| 1968 | Jonas and Donna Salk are divorced. |
| 1970 | Marries Françoise Gilot, world-famous artist and mother of two of Pablo Picasso's children. |
| 1972 | *Man Unfolding*, the first of Salk's philosophical texts is published. *The Survival of the Wisest* follows in 1973. In 1981, his son Jonathan coauthors *World Population and Human Values: A New Reality* with him, and in 1983, *Anatomy of Reality: Merging of Intuition and Reason* is published. |
| 1975 | Steps down from the position of director of the Salk Institute, although he remains in the honorary position of founding director. |
| 1984 | Retires from his lab at the Salk Institute. |
| 1987 | Comes out of retirement to announce that he will begin work on the prospects for controlling the HIV virus and AIDS. |
| 1990 | Announces preliminary success with an HIV vaccine in monkeys and an interest in attempting human tests. |

| | |
|---|---|
| 1992 | Announces that his AIDS research will take a new direction, untried by any other researchers. |
| | Controversy over planned addition to the Salk Institute. |
| | Following announcement by public health officials that no cases of polio have been reported in the Western Hemisphere for more than a year, Salk urges biotechnology leaders to work toward the rapid elimination of polio throughout the world. |

# Glossary

**Adjuvant:** A mineral oil that is added to a vaccine to make it more effective by allowing only small amounts of the vaccine to be absorbed into the blood at a time.

**Antibodies:** The primary weapon of a body's immune system, antibodies are particles in the blood that fight disease by combining with viruses and bacteria and neutralizing them.

**Anti-Semitism:** Prejudice directed against people of Jewish heritage.

**Cell:** The basic structural unit of all living things.

**DNA (deoxyribonucleic acid):** The microscopic material in all cells that tells them how to grow and act. DNA is the operative form of heredity.

**Epidemic:** The outbreak of a disease that affects a whole community.

**Epidemiologist:** A scientist who studies disease as it relates to the community rather than to the individual.

**Evolution:** The gradual development of complex animals and plants from simpler ones through the process of natural selection. In a broader sense, the process by which things build upon what has come before to become more advanced and complex.

**Humanitarian:** Someone who promotes the welfare and health of humankind or anything pertaining to the health and welfare of humankind.

**Immune system:** The body's defense against disease and infection.

**Poliomyelitis:** The scientific name for the disease polio; literally, it means the inflammation of the gray matter of the spinal cord.

**Vaccine:** A substance made of dead or weakened viruses that, when put into a body, causes the body to develop defenses against that disease.

**Viral:** Having to do with viruses.

**Virologist:** A scientist who studies viruses and viral diseases.

**Virulence:** The ability of a virus to cause disease.

**Virus:** A microorganism that causes disease and is dependent upon its host for its existence.

# Bibliography


Alexander, Larry. *The Iron Cradle*. New York: Crowell, 1954. A moving personal narrative by a polio victim.

Carter, Richard. *Breakthrough: The Saga of Jonas Salk*. New York: Trident Press, 1966. A detailed account of the development of the Salk vaccine, the Sabin vaccine, and the surrounding controversy. Strongly partisan in Salk's favor.

Johnson, George. "Once Again a Man with a Mission." *The New York Times Magazine*, November 25, 1990: 57-61. Johnson, an award-winning science writer for *The New York Times*, provides a good critical overview of Salk's personal life and scientific career, from his work on polio to his AIDS research. Emphasizes the controversy in the scientific community with which Salk has had to contend at each stage in his career. Gives many good perspectives from other scientists.

Klein, Aaron. *Trial by Fury*. New York: Charles Scribner's Sons, 1972. A very readable account of the creation of rival polio vaccines and the highly emotional debates over their safety and effectiveness. Considers the place of medical research in the modern world and the ethical and scientific issues at stake in the race to develop a polio vaccine.

Paul, John R. *A History of Poliomyelitis*. New Haven, Conn.: Yale University Press, 1971. A scholarly history of polio from ancient times to the Salk and Sabin vaccines. Includes extensive documentation, and the work relies on a heavy use of medical terminology.

Radetsky, Peter. "Closing in on an AIDS Vaccine." *Discover* 11 (September, 1990): 70-77. An accessible summary of AIDS vaccine work by Salk and other researchers. Vaccine information may be obsolete, but the article provides a good explanation of the problems in developing an AIDS vaccine and outlines some of the leading approaches to a solution.

Rogers, Naomi. *Dirt and Disease: Polio Before FDR*. New Brunswick, N.J.: Rutgers University Press, 1992. This well-researched and readable study deals primarily with the first major polio epidemic in the United States, which took place in the Middle Atlantic states in 1916. Provides valuable background for an understanding of Salk's work with polio.

Salk, Jonas. *Anatomy of Reality: Merging of Intuition and Reason.* New York: Columbia University Press, 1983. In these four demanding works, Salk presents his personal philosophy, founded on a lifetime of reflection on the implications of evolution for every area of human thought and endeavor. The first two books deal largely with scientific ethics. Of the four, *Anatomy of Reality* is the most accessible to general readers, offering a summation of Salk's philosophy.

__________. A Conversation with Jonas Salk." *Psychology Today* 16 (March, 1983): 50-56. In interview form, Salk provides a concrete and personable account of his understanding of humankind, the nature of evolution, and the creative process

__________. *Man Unfolding*. New York: Harper & Row, 1972.

__________. *The Survival of the Wisest*. New York: Harper & Row, 1973.

Salk, Jonas, and Jonathan Salk. *World Population and Human Values: A New Reality*. New York: Harper & Row, 1981.

Smith, Jane. *Patenting the Sun: Polio and the Salk Vaccine*. New York: William Morrow, 1990. This engaging narrative focuses on the children who first took the Salk vaccine, the Polio Pioneers, and how Jonas Salk and the March of Dimes made the vaccine possible. Also provides valuable perspective, placing the development of the polio vaccine in the context of other advances in health and medical technology and the expectations these advances have aroused. Smith's book is the best place to start; in comparison, most other popular treatments of the subject are outdated.

Wilson, John Rowan. *Margin of Safety*. Garden City, N.Y.: Doubleday, 1963. Wilson, a British physician who became the representative in Britain for an American pharmaceutical company engaged in producing polio vaccine, offers a valuable insider's account, but his bias must be taken into account. His

British perspective on what is often considered an American problem is interesting, while his critical and sometimes condescending attitude toward Salk is representative of many in the medical establishment in the 1950's and 1960's.

# Media Resources

*The Body Fights Disease*. Video/16mm film, 13 minutes. 1980. Distributed by Churchill Films. This animated film explores the body's immune system. Briefly discusses bacteria and viruses and explains how immunization works.

*Can You Still Get Polio?* Video, 58 minutes. 1982. Distributed by Coronet/Simon & Schuster Communications. Originally screened in the television series *Nova*, this video discusses the strengths and weaknesses of the killed-virus Salk vaccine and the attenuated-virus Sabin vaccine. Good for both a historical view of the Salk-Sabin controversy and an overview of vaccines and viral diseases.

*Jonas Salk*. 16mm film, 16 minutes. 1969. Distributed by CRM/McGraw-Hill Films. A biographical film focusing on Salk's intense and ultimately successful efforts to develop a safe and effective polio vaccine.

*Jonas Salk: Science and Society*. Video/16mm film, 20 minutes. 1971. Distributed by AIMS Media. Salk talks about the interconnectedness of cancer and other diseases related to failure of the immune system in the context of his work with viruses. He also reflects on the impact of medicine in particular and science in general on the human condition from an ethical standpoint. Offers a good lesson about the immune system as well as an introduction to Salk's distinctive philosophy.

*Salk vs. Polio*. 16mm film, 25 minutes. 1963. Distributed by Wolper Productions. Follows the fight against polio from FDR's founding of the March of Dimes to the Salk vaccine in 1955. The film is more historical than scientific.

*The Science of Hope with Jonas Salk*. Video, 30 minutes. 1992. Distributed by PBS. In this segment from the series *A World of Ideas with Bill Moyers*, Moyers interviews Jonas Salk about the possibilities for a cure for AIDS. Salk speaks engagingly about his own killed-virus research and his theories on how the AIDS crisis fits into the evolutionary history of man and disease. Offers valuable insights into Salk's philosophy as well as the challenge of AIDS research.

*Viruses: Threshold of Life*. Video/16mm film, 13 minutes. 1978. Distributed by Coronet/Simon & Schuster Communications. Discusses viruses and their parasitical nature. Examines the debate as to whether or not viruses are in fact living. Also provides basic instruction in genetics.

**Pioneers**

---

# JONAS SALK

# INDEX